Integrating Spirituality in Health and Social Care

Pe

approaches

WITHDRAWN

Edited by
Wendy Greenstreet
Senior Lecturer
Adult Nursing Studies
Canterbury Christ Church University

Foreword by
Peter Speck

Radcliffe Publishing
Oxford ● Seattle

Radcliffe Publishing Ltd
18 Marcham Road
Abingdon
Oxon OX14 1AA
United Kingdom

www.radcliffe-oxford.com
Electronic catalogue and worldwide online ordering facility.

British Library Cataloguing in Publication Data

A catalogue record for this book is available from the British Library.

ISBN-10: 1 85775 646 0
ISBN-13: 978 1 85775 646 3

Typeset by Advance Typesetting Ltd, Oxford
Printed and bound by TJ International Ltd, Padstow, Cornwall

Contents

Foreword

If you have ever broken a thermometer and tried to pick up the small blobs of mercury, which have scattered all over the floor, you will appreciate how difficult it is to gather them together into a coherent whole. In many ways trying to pull together the various aspects of the word 'spirituality' is equally difficult. The term can prove to be elusive and hard to clarify while, at the same time, being ascribed a centrality of position in the provision of healthcare.[1]

When someone becomes ill their life journey may be diverted into new pathways which will create a variety of anxieties, opportunities, challenges and questions. The questions that arise for people during times of illness will partly relate to causality and they will seek clinical answers. But some questions may relate to the timing and effects of the illness on self and others and lead to a wider discussion of psycho-social-spiritual concerns. Many of the questions focus around 'Why me, why now and what of the future?' I believe that these questions are related to the basic human search for meaning and purpose in our lives and the experiences we have in life. But this is not a vague generalised use of the term meaning. Rather it is the meaning that relates to our very existence on this planet – it is an existential search and concerns 'ultimate' issues. These are not questions we spend a great deal of time pondering when we are busily engaged with our life, but during periods when we are forced aside from our normal routine we have more time to reflect and face some of these ultimate issues. It is for this reason it is important to investigate the relationship between what people believe and the influence those beliefs may, or may not, have on their general health and well-being.

In recent years there has been a growth of interest in the topic as many authors and researchers have tried to define the term and there is now a much wider understanding that spirituality and religion are not necessarily inter-changeable terms.[2] Many people who profess to have developed a spiritual belief system give their belief overt expression through a variety of religious frameworks. Others, however, choose not to and either hold and nurture those beliefs privately or express them without the use of 'religious' language or ritual. There has also been a degree of protectiveness which has discouraged any rigorous research of the concept, until recent years. Within a healthcare setting the rather nebulous nature of the term has caused a degree of confusion for staff who are expected to assess 'spiritual need' and to ensure that those needs are respected and addressed appropriately. The desire for a clear definition is understandable but in the absence of any consensus it is probably more productive to offer 'working descriptions' of how particular authors, policy writers or researchers are using the terms so that the reader can appreciate the stance, and any possible bias, being taken.

I welcome this new publication because Wendy Greenstreet has taken a broad view of the topic and offers a clear overview of the many ways in which the term 'spirituality' is used with healthcare. She also tackles the difficult area of trying to clarify what spirituality might mean for people who are avidly non-religious. One of the strengths of the text is the way in which the theoretical discussion becomes rooted in practical considerations and application which should be of great benefit to those who provide and who receive healthcare in a variety of settings.

Rev Prebendary Peter Speck
Former Healthcare Chaplain
Honorary Senior Research Fellow
King's College London (Palliative Care & Policy)
& Visiting Fellow, Southampton University (Health Psychology)
January 2006

References

1 National Institute for Clinical Excellence (2004) *Guidance on Cancer Services: improving supportive and palliative care for adults with cancer* (N0474); www.nice.org.uk
2 Speck PW (1988) *Being There: pastoral care in time of illness*. SPCK, London.

List of contributors

Hazel Adams
Art Therapist
Blackthorn Trust, Maidstone, Kent

Stephen Clift
Professor of Health Education
Health and Social Welfare Studies and the Sidney De Haan Research Centre
    for Arts and Health
Canterbury Christ Church University

Mo Fiddian
Deputy Services Manager
Heart of Kent Hospice
Aylesford, Kent

Wendy Greenstreet
Senior Lecturer
Adult Nursing Studies
Canterbury Christ Church University

Grenville Hancox MBE
Professor of Music
Department of Music and the Sidney De Haan Research Centre
    for Arts and Health
Canterbury Christ Church University

Derek Mitchell
Visiting Senior Lecturer
Health and Social Welfare Studies
Canterbury Christ Church University

Burkhard Scherer
Senior Lecturer in Religious Studies
Honorary Professor of Indo-Tibetan Buddhism
Canterbury Christ Church University

Sue Timmins
Education Business Manager
East Kent Community Training Alliance

Bons Voors
Counsellor (MBACP)
Blackthorn Trust, Maidstone, Kent

Rev Professor Stephen G Wright MBE
Faculty of Health and Social Care
St Martin's College, Carlisle
Chairman, The Sacred Space Foundation, Cumbria
Editor of *Spirituality and Health International*

Acknowledgements

My thanks go to all contributors whose work has enriched the creation of this book. Thanks also go to Yvonne Hill, Head of Department, Adult Nursing Studies, and Sue Holmes (Professor), Director of Research and Development, Faculty of Health and Social Care, both at Canterbury Christ Church University for their support and encouragement with this project.

Particular thanks must go to my husband, Graham, and my son and daughter, Ben and Sophie, for their love and forbearance throughout.

Introduction

Wendy Greenstreet

The scope of this book is to consider the role of spirituality as a core component of health and social care. As a generic text it is not focused on any particular profession or practice, but rather provides an introduction to this complex concept. All health and social care professionals include 'care' as a central component of their daily work, albeit from a different disciplinary perspective and at varied intensity in relation to technical practice. This guide is, therefore, an introduction to spirituality and claims only to encourage readers to take a step over the threshold of enquiry into an aspect of care that is irreducible and difficult to quantify, and so risk a discomfort of thought that might be seen to be incongruent with the empirical focus of today's evidence-based practice.

The book comprises four sections. The first explores available research and published literature that helps us understand what is meant by spirituality and what this may mean in relation to health and social care provision. It provides a somewhat theoretical and esoteric start, but I would encourage perseverance as it outlines a foundation of knowledge that underpins the later practice-focused discussion.

The first chapter begins by owning that any attempt to conceptualise what is in fact abstract, such as spirituality, results in a contrived reality that is to some extent an illusion. Moving on, the term 'person' is considered. Frequently used to convey a sense of value in itself,[1] the term 'person' is affirmed in the practical and altruistic drives to make provision for care for those persons who are unwell or challenged by the circumstances they find themselves in. Giving some consideration to what we mean by 'person' is helpful in clarifying each profession's claim to provide care; their focus, boundaries and shared practice. More particularly, it should convey an awareness of what constitutes spirituality as part of the person as an individual and reflected in spirituality as a perspective of holistic care. Meaning, relationship and a 'sense of becoming' are some examples of consensus in published literature of the characteristics of spirituality. Spirituality is integrated with other perspectives of person and it can, perhaps, be difficult to understand the difference between a spiritual and a psychological need. The term 'spirituality' seems to be used by cultures that are English speaking and its interpretation across world religions varies. Age and maturation seem to potentially contribute to a strengthened spirituality.

The second chapter considers how the analytical ambience of the twentieth century has seen the glorification of quantifiable scientific knowledge at the expense of the qualitative 'art' of care. The historical association of caring for the sick within religious vocation contributes to confusion in understanding the concept of spirituality and a tendency for it to be equated with religion. In an increasingly secular society this results in a potential neglect of spiritual care. The emergence of a 'holistic' person-centred model of care that challenges reductionist philosophy describes spirituality as a component of multidimensional care. This model demands a shift in focus from efficiency and the task of care to authentic relationship in which the professional is personally able to contribute to care. The polarisation of spirituality as religious, sacred or secular is challenged as being artificial and the suggestion made that it is better reflected as 'a family of different yet connected meanings'[2] (p.237).

In considering spiritual wellbeing and spiritual distress, the focus of the book begins to shift more towards practice contexts. Health is considered as a balance between human control and spirituality. Spiritual wellness is discussed and associated with a striving for growth, while spiritual distress is related to meaninglessness. Spiritual need is depicted as a continuum between these two states. In supporting others in spiritual need we must first know ourselves well and consider our own spiritual stance, and the reasons why this is important are considered. Spiritual intelligence is said to provide us with a means of achieving wellbeing. However, how are we to assess spiritual need, does this require 'spiritual assessment' or gathering information concerning a patient's spirituality?[3]

The second section of the book is practice focused. It is important not to contrive spiritual care as an objective reality or prescribe it as a requirement by all those within care contexts. Spiritual care can be classified as an activity that professionals can 'do' for their patients, or support offered within an established rapport. Activities considered are religious rituals, 'New Age' and creative therapy. 'Doing' also involves referral to appropriate others when we reach the boundaries of our ability to provide spiritual care. As an integral part of, rather than an adjunct to, care, spiritual support is largely delivered through a professional client/patient relationship that can be described as covenantal, based on mutual sharing.[4] This style of relationship is not easy for professionals ensconced in the objectivity that professionalisation promotes. It requires both confidence and experience in communicating, particularly through active listening,[5] and the courage to stay with vulnerability that might remind us of our own. In listening and presence, professionals open themselves to client/patient storytelling. It is often through narrative and metaphor that spiritual matters are expressed. Storytelling may seem repetitive and confused but may reflect client/patient review of their own biography in attempting to find meaning in their current difficulty. In 'clearing away the clutter'[6] (p.23) by using simple questions, such as 'what do you want me to do for you?' or 'what do you seek?', professional carers can participate sensitively in helpful dialogue.

Hope is universally accepted as a positive quality and its absence linked to despair. Chapter 5 explores hope in relation to spirituality. Whether hope is general or concerned with particular hopes, it is influenced by cultural understanding of this concept. Tools that measure hope are limited in the same way as tools that assess spirituality. However, theory that helps the reader understand hope as a process and outlines strategies that promote hope provides useful guidelines that might help in the delivery of spiritual care. Illustrative case studies exemplify this.

The final chapter of this section considers the spiritual context of work and the importance and sources of support for those professionals involved in spiritual care. Relationships at work are described as mirroring the nature of the corporate body. Work devoid of meaning is dispiriting and results in poorer performance and attendance. Language transmits conscious and unconscious signals that may influence the way we feel about work, for example when 'people' are 'resources'.

Options for making work more soulful, which do not have to be complicated or expensive, are suggested.

The third section provides robust religious and philosophical comment and ends with the practical implications that religious and cultural diversity might present in practice. Starting with the history and philosophy behind the term 'religion', the discussion leads on to consider 'religion' in relation to the broader term 'spirituality'. Conventional classification of religion, for example, into Eastern or Western tradition, is reviewed and an alternative grouping suggested. This is a comparative classification that compares religions of faith with those of experience. The significance of each is then considered in relation to ill health.

In a serious attempt to make existentialist philosophy accessible to health and social care professionals, the works of Sartre and Heidegger are used to convey a notion of selfhood and being with others, which epitomises the style of authentic relationship that is the vehicle for providing spiritual care. This style of authentic relationship is advocated as being appropriate for provision of the spiritual dimension of care in all care settings.

In a multicultural population, care that acknowledges and is sensitive to the diversity of religious practice and cultural identity promotes spiritual wellbeing. The importance of raising the awareness of professional carers is discussed, along with the application of knowledge of cultural and religious variance to clients/patients. Practical issues such as diet, physical examination and specific cultural and religious requirements in terminal care are considered.

The final section considers creative options for care that potentially extend consciousness and an awareness of transcendence or help establish meaning in difficulty. Rudolf Steiner's anthroposophical philosophy underpins the Blackthorn project. Its establishment within a National Health Service general practice demonstrates how the creative can enhance the conventional provision of care in a very real way. Chapter 10 introduces Steiner's work, particularly anthroposophical medicine. Biographical counselling is described as an example of individual therapy, as well as a variety of group activities. Art as therapy is also anthroposophical in that it illustrates another of Blackthorn's creative options. Starting with a historical outline that demonstrates a shift in how art has been viewed over time, this chapter goes on to illustrate the benefits of art by the use of case studies. The final chapter considers music and its contribution to healthcare. Research on spirituality, music and health are considered and examples of organisations that bring music to healthcare described. Music-thanatology has particular relevance to spirituality for those who are dying, but the chapter closes by acknowledging caution in making assumptions about music's contribution to spiritual care.

References

1 Habgood J (1998) *Being a Person, Where Faith and Science Meet.* Hodder and Stoughton, London.
2 van Leeuwen R, Cusvellar B (2004) Nursing competencies for spiritual care. *Journal of Advanced Nursing.* **48**(3): 234–46.
3 Pierpont JH (2003) Spiritual Assessment. *Social Work.* **48**(4): 562–3.
4 Bradshaw A (1994) *Lighting the Lamp: the spiritual dimension of nursing care.* Scutari Press, Harrow.

5 Carson VB (1989) *Spiritual Dimensions of Nursing Practice.* Saunders, Philadelphia, PA.
6 Guenther M (1992) *Holy Listening, The Art of Spiritual Direction.* Darton, Longman and Todd, London.

Exploring the concept of spirituality

CHAPTER 1

Clarifying the concept

Wendy Greenstreet

Introduction

This chapter introduces the concept of spirituality by exploring the views expressed in published literature. Dictionary definitions are limited, describing the term 'spirituality' as a derivative of the word 'spiritual', which means 'relating to, or affecting the human spirit as opposed to material or physical things', or 'relating to religion or religious belief'.[1] The need to express spirituality as a concept rather than a term reflects our having to use imagination to help us with what is both difficult to understand and explain. A succinct contemporary dictionary definition, for example, suggests that a concept is 'something conceived'.[1] A more detailed, contemplative description of the term 'concept'[2] starts by exploring our need to understand reality by using ideas. For ideas that are nebulous rather than physical or concrete, we create concepts. To understand the reality that is represented by the concept we seek to define it and so give what are nebulous boundaries. Consequently, the conceptual knowledge that results gives us an intellectual grasp of what is nebulous, that is to some extent based on an illusion. This is true of spirituality.

The concept of spirituality is derived from human reflection and imagination as well as logical reasoning.[3] It is particularly intangible and eludes true definition, needing to be grounded in a specific context if any attempt to describe it is to be helpful. In exploring the concept of spirituality as it is seen within health and social care, this chapter attempts to enable professional practitioners to understand how spirituality constitutes a perspective of care. This exploration starts with a consideration of spirituality as a component of being a person, and then interprets what is meant by the concept, its boundaries and preconditions.[4] Consideration will also be given to spirituality and faith as a lifespan issue, and the need for a common language of spirituality among professional carers.

Spirituality as a component of being a person

All persons are embodied in a physical form, but the human body as an entity does not constitute a person. Habgood[5] uses an example of ethical dilemma to explore the characteristics that might describe the parameters of being a person. Belonging, both psychologically and socially, is central to being a person. Who we are is seated in our experience of our cultural environment. Communicating with others contributes to our growth and the growth of those we communicate with, 'we need to *be* something before we can properly relate' (p.117), but 'we can only become something in that we *do* relate to others' (p.118). The use of the term 'individual' in relation to a person is also considered and reference made to two interpretations, both of which are worthy of consideration in relation to health and social care. The first of these is individual as indivisible, referring to 'that which cannot be divided into parts without destroying its essential nature' (p.60). Individual is also a person with a distinct, separate existence from all other persons who collectively constitute humanity. The individual is differentiated from others symbolically by having a name. A higher level of consciousness accounts for personal awareness of the self as human and the human condition ending in death.[6] Becoming a person is a process, as is its 'slow dissolution ... through illness or old age'[5] (p.28).

The presence of spirituality as part of personhood is seldom discussed until it is challenged or dislocated.[7] Whereas the physical aspects of person can be seen and the psychological and social acted out in behaviours that can be observed, spirituality may remain covert. Therefore the indivisible nature of a person, as an individual, may be portrayed with spirituality at the core of an integrated 'whole' (Figure 1.1) in that the physical, psychological and social aspects of the person overlap.

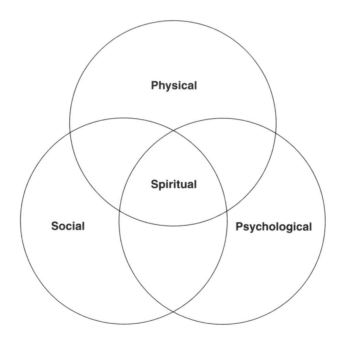

Figure 1.1 Spirituality as a component of being a person; individual as indivisible.

Inclusion of the physical-spiritual, psycho-spiritual and the social-spiritual (Figure 1.2) aspects of a person still leaves spirituality depicted as the 'inner' hidden presence implied by Cobb.[7]

The implicit nature of an inner spirituality makes explicit definition of the concept difficult. Wright and Sayre-Adams,[8] see 'each human being as part of the universe which is a dynamic web of interconnected and interrelated events, none of which function in isolation' (p.9). This perhaps reflects the alternative view of the individual as a named person within a greater collective humanity. Definition of

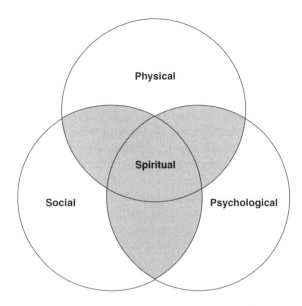

Figure 1.2 Spiritual, physical-spiritual, socio-spiritual and psycho-spiritual components of being a person.

a concept as nebulous as spirituality within such an encompassing view of a person is also difficult.

What is spirituality?

Culliford[9] describes spirituality as an essentially unifying link between the deeply personal and the universal. The inner, hidden presence and universal web of spirituality are thus conveyed as two parts of the same phenomenon. McColl,[10] however, offers a different and thought-provoking view. She differentiates between spirituality, which is a human characteristic, and spirit, which is something that exists independently. Spirit is incorporated in our lives according to our ability to experience it. The ability to recognise this experience is our spirituality and the experience itself is one of transcendence. Although we may use the senses, emotions and intellect to interpret transcendent experiences as being, for example, those of awe, mystery or even fear, there is no language to describe the experience of transcendence, so we rely on symbols and metaphors to try and convey a sense of the indefinable.[11]

Literature reviews[12,13] and analyses of the concept of spirituality[14,15] have not revealed, or resulted in the creation of, a universally accepted definition of spirituality. However, there is some consensus in published literature about the attributes/characteristics of this concept.

The first of these is that every person has a spiritual dimension,[16] although the description of the form this takes varies. McColl[10] gives examples of literature that suggest spirituality is the essence of self, but argues that a shared spirit experienced through transcendence, rather than one possessed by the self encouraging introspection, avoids a distorted emphasis on how the world relates to self and a better perception of self in the context of a grander scheme. Ultimate beliefs and values stem from the spiritual dimension of the person,[17] and their outward expression is individual, shaped by factors such as life experience and culture.[18] For example, those who value environmental preservation would live in a style that reflected a 'green' philosophy, or those who had explored various religious doctrines might find faith in a 'God' and live according to the requirements of that faith.

Published comment generally accepts that the terms 'spirituality' and 'religion' are not synonymous. Heriot[19] differentiates between spirituality and religion by describing spirituality as a broader notion, an 'umbrella' under which the means of fulfilling spiritual needs is found. Speck[18] describes religion as a system of faith and worship that expresses an underlying spirituality; this explains how religion can be found beneath Heriot's[19] spiritual umbrella as an example of a means of fulfilling spiritual need rather than doing so exclusively.[20] In exploring the psychology of religion at the beginning of the twentieth century, James[21] differentiated between personal and institutional religion, considering men's personal experiences of 'whatever they may consider the divine' (p.31) the backbone of the world's religious life, and that 'Churches, when once established, live at second-hand upon tradition' (p.30). This person(al) dimension has been a common element to both religion and the concept of spirituality.[12] For those whose spirituality is not related to religion, for example an atheist who denies the existence of God, or an agnostic who is unsure of God's existence, the beliefs that become the driving force in their lives may be a strong belief in significant relationships, or self-chosen values or goals.[22] Dawson,[23] for example, explains:

> In spite of my professed atheism, I cannot dispel the idea that perhaps the spiritual outlook on the world has some deep and unrecognised evolutionary benefit, and that our present fascination with, and mystification by, positivistic naturalism, the scientific outlook, may constitute a fatal aberration. (p.287)

The search for meaning, life's purpose and the significance of existence are commonly discussed in describing spirituality.[17,24] Making sense of life situations is frequently significant in health and social care contexts. This search within particular life events often takes the form of questioning, asking why?[25–27] For example:

- Why me?
- What have I done to deserve this?
- Why now?
- Why do I have to suffer?

Goddard[28] classifies ultimate questions according to focus (Table 1.1).

Table 1.1 Classification of ultimate questions[28]

Eschatological	Death and afterlife
Noumenological	Intuition and mind
Thaumatological	Miracles
Ontological	Being

McColl[10] explains a reciprocal relationship between meaning and spirituality in that spirituality invests activities with meaning, and meaningful activities express spirituality. She also differentiates between meaning *in* life, as a lower order of meaning that refers to specific activities and their meanings, and the meaning *of* life, as a higher order of meaning that refers to the meaning of one's whole life. Examples of sources of meaning in life are work, personal gain or relationships with significant others.[29] Some might find meaning in a religion, but religious philosophies may interpret meaning as an attribute of spirituality in different ways. For example, MacLaren[30] explains that although individuals belonging to a Judeo-Christian culture might ask ultimate questions regarding the circumstances they find themselves in, Mahayana Buddhists attempt to reach a state of 'meaning-free-ness' by remaining open and responsive to enable passion to become compassion and intellect wisdom.

Connectedness or connecting is a frequently used term in describing spirituality.[3,17] This refers to a variety of forms of relationship: the intrapersonal or connecting with self; the interpersonal or connecting with others; and transpersonal, which describes connecting with a higher power/God and the environment. These differing relationships also have a history of being described in a two-dimensional fashion; intrapersonal and interpersonal having a horizontal dimension and the transpersonal as vertical.[31] This multiplicity of relationships once again reflects spirituality as an inner quality of self that is expressed and experienced within the immediate world that we share with others and also as part of a larger world/universe. The nature of love within these relationships differs. Conditional love comes most easily to man and is associated with human 'needs'.[32] It is prompted by attractive qualities or what others have to offer. Unconditional love is associated with a person's source of transcendence and is considered a more spiritually fulfilling love. Unconditional love is also known as agape. Campbell[33] considers professional ethics to be underpinned by the demands of unconditional love, to love equally and without partiality. He describes caring within a professional context as an example of self-transcendence. Transcendence as an experience and appreciation of a dimension beyond the self that expands self-boundaries is described as a significant attribute of spirituality.[10,34] Dawson[23] refers to different interpretations of transcendence as reflecting that even secular thinkers have 'a deep and abiding desire to move beyond the mundane to a grander eschatological vision' (p.288). His references include Reich's (1970) transcendence as personal liberation, Bloch's (1970) Marxist transcendence as future, and Jung (1933, 1935) and Laing's (1960, 1967) transcendence as self-realisation or self-creation. Transcendence reflects humanity's capacity to cope with unsolvable problems. In this way, struggle can lead to growth. Sermabeikian[35] uses the following quote to explain this:

> This transcendence of the individual's personal problems reveals itself as a raising of the level of consciousness. A loftier and wider interest comes into view, and through this broadening of the horizon the insoluble problem loses its urgency. It is not logically solved in its own terms but pales before a new and stronger vital direction. It is not repressed and made unconscious but simply appears in a new light and so becomes itself different. (p.181)

The association of spirituality with an unfolding of life is referred to as 'becoming'. Who we are and how we 'know' come from reflection and experience.[17] Hope is a component of becoming in enabling creativity and a sense of future. So is the ability to forgive ourselves, being able to live with our 'flaws',[36] and is particularly well addressed by the following:

> There is a progression from trust in the acceptance by others of all the things in ourselves that we regret into a faith in forgiveness, where we at last believe that they have no more power to hurt us or anyone else. We cannot alter what has happened or what we have done, but we can come to believe that the meaning of the past can be changed. From this comes the ability to forgive ourselves. This may never be expressed in words on either side but the quality of the ensuing peace is unmistakable.[37] (p.55)

Defining spirituality in a way that is comprehensive in including the range of characteristics that constitute the concept, without implying religious bias or exclusion of religion, or in advocating a singularly secular statement, verges on the impossible. However, a popular choice of definition in published literature that conveys the concept as wider than religion without excluding religion or making it requisite is:

> A quality that goes beyond religious affiliation, that strives for inspirations, reverence, awe, meaning and purpose, even in those who do not believe in God. The spiritual dimension tries to be in harmony with the universe, strives for answers about the infinite and comes into focus when the person faces emotional stress, physical illness and death.[38] (p.259)

McSherry[39] suggests this definition reflects spirituality as subjective, unique, universal and mysterious, and, at the same time, as complex, personal and sensitive. Culliford[9] also supports this definition and suggests that mental illness should be added to the definition's closing list of circumstances that heighten a spiritual focus. However, it does have its critics. Bash[40] suggests this definition attempts to answer the question of what is spirituality by using 'secular terms but using language and thought forms to do with the transcendent' and 'so offers a sort of religionless religion' that 'is a muddle' (p.12). It also fails to convey the sense of struggle that can be part of the spiritual focus of those who find themselves in health and social care contexts. Definition is the conventional starting point for both analysis and evaluation of a concept.[4] The difficulty in defining the concept of spirituality accounts for a lack of clarity and an enduring sense of confusion about the response to the question 'what is spirituality?'

Boundaries, preconditions and outcomes

Concepts that pertain to aspects of a person inevitably have murky boundaries because, although they are useful intellectual constructs for us to understand humanity, they are not real in the sense that a person is a gestalt whole, being more than the sum of conceptual parts. The blurring of boundaries of the conceptual physical, psychological, social and spiritual parts of a person can be represented in the overlap of these concepts (Figure 1.2). One of the most controversial boundaries identified in published literature is determining how psychological and spiritual dimensions of person differ.[41]

Benjamin and Looby[42] cite Rogers' (1980) and Maslow's (1971) work in suggesting that the use of the term 'self-actualisation' reflects the nature of spirituality in their theories. Both psychologists are said to believe that personal autonomy, self-acceptance, open communication and interaction, and the freedom to make choices are characteristics of a self-actualised person. Similarly, reference is made to Maslow's assertion that individuals who reach the peak of self-actualisation are transcendent self-actualisers who have a holistic perspective of the world and a natural tendency towards co-operative action. These descriptions of self-actualisation collectively share all forms of connectedness that are characteristic of spirituality, and so self-actualisation may be considered representative of the psycho-spiritual aspect of self (Figure 1.2). This does not mean that self-actualisation alone is equal to spirituality. In referring to 'the peak of self-actualisation', Maslow infers that it is possible to arrive at this state, that the striving for self-actualisation that Rogers refers to is in fact a destination. However, spirituality is better depicted as a journey, an ongoing search[43] and a dynamic sense of becoming.[17] Spirituality is also construed to be an aspect of every person, but only the minority of persons are likely to achieve the altruistic heights of peak self-actualisation.

As a constituent of being a person, psychologists are interested in spirituality as a dimension of personality and its contribution to intrinsic motivation. This is not to confuse psychological motivational theory with spirituality. It is a different dimension and is therefore able to bring a novel element to the field of psychology in its focus on how individuals construct meaning in their lives.[6]

The use of the term 'spirituality' in relation to healthcare seems to be bounded by cultures that are English speaking and rarely used in Catholic or profoundly religious countries.[44,45] Within the Chinese culture in Taiwan, the term 'thought' is used to describe psycho-spiritual dimensions and the term 'mind' to describe psycho-social-spiritual dimensions. However, in an attempt to develop culturally relevant palliative care provision Chao *et al.*[46] explored the essence of spirituality in six terminally ill Taiwanese patients. Participants in the study included those of Buddhist, Protestant and Catholic faiths. The patterns that emerged (Table 1.2) were comparable with the previous discussion of the varied forms of connectedness as

Table 1.2 Essence of spirituality in Taiwanese study[46]

Patterns	*Themes*
Communion with self	• self-identity – discovery of authentic self • wholeness – despite human contradictions • inner peace – negotiating conflicts for self-reconciliation
Communion with others	• love – caring but not over-attachment to others • reconciliation – to forgive and to be forgiven
Communion with nature	• inspiration – the resonance of the marvellous beauty of nature • creativity – conceiving imaginatively
Communion with higher being	• faithfulness – keeping the trust dependably • hope – claiming possibilities • gratitude – giving thanks and embracing grace

part of spirituality defined within healthcare (see above), reflecting communion with self, others, nature and a higher being. Similarly, themes included discovery of the authentic self as comparable with 'becoming' as well as forgiveness and hope (Table 1.2).

Although only a small study, it does demonstrate difference in relation to use of the terminology of spirituality and yet overlap in essence of understanding across English and non-English speaking cultures of this dimension of person. Markham[44] explains that although not all religions recognise the term spirituality, most practise activities surrounding prayer and meditation that take on the characteristics of this term. Alternative understandings of spirituality vary in focus across different religions (Table 1.3) and also 'alternative accounts' of these understandings are to be found within the interpretation of each religion[44] (p.74).

Table 1.3 Examples of Alternative Understandings of Spirituality[44]

Islam	Spirituality as extinction of the self
Judaism	Discovering spirituality in the mundane
Hinduism	Spirituality as the discovery of the real self
Buddhism	Spirituality within the ethical

Therefore, collectively, these religious 'spiritualities' might be considered potentially boundless. Regardless of terminology used to describe the spiritual dimension of person, what is universally agreed is that it is a complex phenomenon.[44]

The fundamental precondition of the concept of spirituality is its 'humanness' (Swinton 1999, cited[47]). Humanity's relation to the universe is described as a worldview. Spirituality, in dealing with ultimate meaning, is closely linked to worldviews.[17] Professional world-views are a precondition of the concept of spirituality in health and social care. In nursing, for example, although there are many conceptual models. Fawcett[48] believes that these only reflect two world-views. Spirituality is 'seen' in each world-view but described differently.

For example, Martsolf[17] describes one of these as a reciprocal interaction worldview; humans are comprised of dimensions that are viewed in the context of the whole. Interactions between humans and their environments are reciprocal, with change occurring continuously or in response to threats to survival. Spirituality within this world-view is seen as a dimension of the person that interacts with other parts of the individual in a holistic way. This is only an example of describing a world-view and individuals will each have their own world-view. To contribute to spiritual care, professional carers need a world-view that includes spirituality.

The outcomes associated with the concept of spirituality within health and social care contexts are either the presence of spiritual health or spiritual wellbeing or its absence in spiritual distress. These are discussed in Chapter 3.

Spirituality and faith as a lifespan issue

Courtenay[49] considers the process of becoming a person as one of personal and faith development. In doing so, he is not equating faith with religion, but uses

Fowler's view of faith as a universal mode that transcends religion. Faith is therefore seen as:

> people's evolved and enhancing ways of experiencing self, others and world (as they construct them) as related to and affected by the ultimate conditions of existence (as they construct them) and of shaping their lives' purposes and meanings, trusts and loyalties, in light of the character of being, value and power determining the ultimate conditions of existence (as grasped in their operative images-conscious and unconscious-of them). (Fowler 1981, cited,[49] p.159)

Courtenay[49] outlines the outcome of Fowler's research in describing the potential for the development of faith across the lifespan as having six stages (Table 1.4). The roots of this model are described as eclectic, drawing on psychological development theory, particularly cognitive (Piaget), moral (Kohlberg) and personality (Erikson) staged models. Socialisation, philosophical and theological theory are also utilised. This staged model of faith has much to offer in understanding the development of spirituality across the lifespan.

Table 1.4   Fowler's six stages of faith development

Stage	Faith
1 Early childhood	Intuitive–projective
2 School years	Mythic–literal
3 Adolescence	Synthetic–conventional
4 Young adulthood	Individuative–reflective
5 Mid-life and beyond	Conjunctive
6 No age range	Universalising

Spirituality in health and social care contexts is similar to the concept of faith described by Fowler. Both are wider concepts than religion but acknowledge the potential role of religion. However, the role of religion within each concept differs. Within the concept of spirituality, religion might fulfil the needs of the human spirit but others achieve fulfilment of these needs without any notion of deity.[20] Fowler divorces religion from faith development in making the point that faith transcends religion and so describes faith in descriptive stages rather than prescriptive religious requirement. Fowler believed faith to be concerned with the 'making, maintenance and transformation of human meaning' (Fowler 1986, cited,[50] p.119). However, he does state that religious content is probably essential for moving from stage 5 to stage 6 in faith development. This suggests that secular spirituality would not enable a person to develop universalising faith as described by Fowler. In reality, so few persons achieve stage 6 of faith development that this difference is unlikely to impact consideration of faith development as a means of understanding the development of spirituality across the lifespan.

Stages of faith are attached to periods of life and so reliant on age and maturation. Spirituality in children is dependent on their developmental stage.[51] Smith and McSherry[52] make reference to Fowler's stages of faith in their consideration of spiritual awareness in children. Fowler's early stages of faith are undifferentiated.

Faith in pre- and early school years is therefore intuitive and filled with uninhibited imagination. Concrete thinking is the stimulus to move the child on to literal interpretations of story and explanation during school years. Fowler's early stages of faith development suggest that a comprehensive understanding of child development and associated cognitive and linguistic skills provides the key for professional carers to understand and access an awareness of a child's spirituality.

Contradictions in belief that demand reflection move the child on to stage 3 of faith in adolescence. This stage is about conformity and Fowler believes many adults do not move beyond this. Faith requires commitment, and adults have commitments to family, job and community. As clashes and contradictions between valued authorities provide the stimulus to move individuals on to stage 4, some might not choose to move and so grow in faith. Courtenay[49] quotes the following and this can be taken as an example:

> Most adults are richly enmeshed in a fabric of relationships which hold them as they are, and many of their friends and relations do not wish them to change ... Sometimes it is just plain simpler to stay right where they are, or at least to appear that way. (Daloz 1988, cited,[49] p.165)

In these circumstances the fabric of relationships provides an overarching sense of meaning that makes it possible to sustain difficult commitments as an act of faith. Here, professional carers need to support an adult person in their decision regarding change.

Those who move on to stages 4 and 5 of faith development shift from reflection on the tension between opposites, such as individual and group identity, to an ability in mid-life and beyond to see both sides of an issue, to be open to paradox and contradiction. Maturation sees a potential shift of emphasis in energy expenditure from sexuality to spirituality.[53] MacKinlay[50] suggests that examining spirituality in the context of wisdom in later life indicates an increased tolerance of ambiguity and awareness of the contradictory nature of reality, a deeper search for meaning and a shift from external sources to internal regulation. She advocates that the relationship between professional carers and older people should be one of partnership in which the considerable wisdom of those in later life, and their ability to be involved in complex problem solving related to their wellbeing, would acknowledge spirituality as a dimension in older people.

Few achieve the sixth stage of universalising faith in which there is a lack of concern for the self and a vision to transform the world. Fowler gives Gandhi and Martin Luther King as examples of those who have achieved this level of faith.

Stages of faith are hierarchical, moving from earlier undifferentiated to the later complex, flexible and comprehensive. Stages cannot be skipped and the sequence cannot be reversed unless there is mental (cognitive) or emotional (affective) deterioration. McSherry and Cash[54] point out that contemporary definitions of spirituality in healthcare include the notion of functioning intellect and, therefore, exclude a large number of individuals who have neurological or cognitive impairment and so are unable to intellectualise or reason. Here, Fowler's model of faith offers some understanding of how the spirituality of these individuals may be described. Congenital cognitive or affective impairment would mean that an individual's faith is more likely to be undifferentiated and, depending on the degree of impairment, would be described as stage 1 or stage 2 of faith. Similarly, if an adult becomes cognitively or affectively impaired, their faith development may be reversed and they could revert to an undifferentiated stage of faith. This may help professionals understand spirituality in relation to care of neurologically or cognitively impaired clients/patients.

Life crises and dilemmas can result in a transition to the next stage of faith or intransigence, in the same way as ill health, loss and suffering are described as resulting in spiritual growth or distress. Faith development, like spirituality, is dynamic, an ongoing process that means a person can form and reform their way of being in and seeing the world throughout their lifespan.

Lifespan development of spirituality, like faith, is about potentiality. As a seed present in all human beings it may remain largely dormant, but many will see some germination and evidence of growth, and the few achieve altruistic proportions.

Language and spirituality

Habgood[5] points out that language is never a private possession, we know ourselves through the medium of a shared culture which, in part, involves the active creation, redefinition and reorientation of the space within which experience is shared. Health services, dominated by language of the marketplace, need to reintroduce 'spirituality' into the language of nurses[55] and other professional carers. Nolan and Crawford[55] believe rhetoric is the way to create meaning and that the rhetoric of spirituality is needed to ensure that the spiritual is valued alongside the scientific. Education is a means of raising professional carers' awareness of spirituality and promoting confidence in dealing with spirituality in practice.[56] Nevertheless, the professional language of rhetoric can open up a gap between theory and practice. McSherry and Watson[57] argue that education is generating an awareness of an aspect of care not fully understood by the general population. This means that professionals should not assume that a common language of spirituality is recognisable by all patients. The need is for a common language of spirituality among professional carers. Achieving an awareness of the parameters of this aspect of care should help the professional in the interpretation of need rather than expecting clients/patients to categorise their need as spiritual. For example, does a client/patient expressing questions that search for meaning, asking the whys of their current circumstances, need to have a common language of spirituality with the professional? It is for the professional to identify the nature of this need as spiritual and provide the appropriate support or refer to another who can.

Conclusion

The dual interpretation of the term 'individual' reflects the nature of spirituality as a component of being a person. The interpretation of individual as an indivisible 'whole' is complemented by that of the named individual as one of a collective humanity. Spirituality in the former is hidden, an inner potential or presence, and in the latter reflected as an outer interconnected and interrelated aspect of person as part of the universe. Each person has a spiritual dimension that may be expressed in religion, existential meaning, through relationship(s), and in hope and forgiveness as part of 'becoming'. The boundaries of the concept of spirituality are murky and its core difficult to define, but its relation to 'humanness' and humanity's relation to the universe are fundamental. Faith is linked to spirituality and spiritual development to age and maturation. The rhetoric of spirituality is needed to establish its value as an aspect of care in an ambience dominated by empirical measurement and evidence-based practice.

References

1   Pearsall J (ed.) (2001) *Concise Oxford Dictionary.* Oxford University Press, Oxford.
2   Merton T (1951) *The Ascent to Truth.* Hollis and Carter, London.
3   Reed PG (1992) An emerging paradigm for the investigation of spirituality in nursing. *Research in Nursing & Health.* **15**: 349–57.
4   Morse J, Mitcham C, Hupcey JE *et al.* (1996) Criteria for concept evaluation. *Journal of Advanced Nursing.* **24**(2): 385–90.
5   Habgood J (1998) *Being a Person.* Hodder and Stoughton, London.
6   Piedmont R (2004) Spiritual transcendence as a predictor of psychosocial outcome from an outpatient substance abuse program. *Psychology of Addictive Behaviours.* **18**(3): 213–22.
7   Cobb M (2001) *The Dying Soul.* Open University Press, Buckingham.
8   Wright SG, Sayre-Adams J (2000) *Sacred Space, Right Relationship and Spirituality in Healthcare.* Churchill Livingstone, Edinburgh.
9   Culliford L (2002) Spirituality and clinical care: spiritual values and skills are increasingly recognised as necessary aspects of clinical care. *British Medical Journal.* **325**(7378): 1434–5.
10 McColl AM (2000) Spirit, occupation and disability. *Canadian Journal of Occupational Therapy.* **67**(4): 217–28.
11 Stanworth R (2004) *Recognizing Spiritual Needs in People Who Are Dying.* Oxford University Press, Oxford.
12 Emblen JD (1992) Religion and spirituality defined according to current use in nursing literature. *Journal of Professional Nursing.* **8**(1): 41–7.
13 Dyson J, Cobb M, Forman D (1997) The meaning of spirituality: a literature review. *Journal of Advanced Nursing.* **26**(6): 1183–8.
14 Tanyi R (2002) Towards clarification of the meaning of spirituality. *Journal of Advanced Nursing.* **39**(5): 500–9.
15 Delgado D (2005) A discussion of the concept of spirituality. *Nursing Science Quarterly.* **18**(2): 157–62.
16 Stoter D (1995) *Spiritual Aspects of Health Care.* Mosby, London.
17 Martsolf D (1998) The concept of spirituality in nursing theories: differing world-views and the extent of focus. *Journal of Advanced Nursing.* **27**(2): 294–303.
18 Speck P (1998) The meaning of spirituality in illness. In: Cobb M, Robshaw V (eds) *The Spiritual Challenge of Health Care.* Churchill Livingstone, Edinburgh.
19 Heriot CS (1992) Spirituality and ageing. *Holistic Nursing Practice.* **7**(1): 22–31.
20 Greenstreet W (1999) Teaching spirituality in nursing: a literature review. *Nurse Education Today.* **19**: 649–58.
21 James W (1982) *The Varieties of Religious Experience.* Penguin, Middlesex.
22 Burnard P (1988) The spiritual needs of atheists and agnostics. *Professional Nurse.* **4**: 130–2.
23 Dawson PJ (1997) A reply to Goddard's 'spirituality as integrative energy'. *Journal of Advanced Nursing.* **25**(2): 282–9.
24 Narayanasamy A (2004) Commentary. *Journal of Advanced Nursing.* **45**(5): 462–4.
25 Speck P (1992) Nursing the soul. *Nursing Times.* **88**(23): 22.
26 Twycross R (1999) *Introducing Palliative Care.* Radcliffe Medical Press, Oxford.
27 Peberdy A (2000) Spiritual care of dying people. In: Dickenson D, Johnson M, Samson Katz J (eds) *Death, Dying and Bereavement.* Open University Press/Sage, London.
28 Goddard NC (2000) A response to Dawson's critical analysis of 'spirituality as "integrative energy"'. *Journal of Advanced Nursing.* **31**(4): 968–79.
29 Oldnall A (1996) A critical analysis of nursing: meeting the spiritual needs of patients. *Journal of Advanced Nursing.* **23**(1): 138–44.

30 MacLaren J (2004) A kaleidoscope of understandings: spiritual nursing in a multi-faith society. *Journal of Advanced Nursing.* **45**(5): 457–62.
31 Moberg D (ed.) (1979) *Spiritual Well-being: sociological perspectives.* University Press of America, Washington DC.
32 Lewis CS (1971) *The Four Loves.* Fontana, Glasgow.
33 Campbell AV (1984) *Moderated Love, A Theology of Professional Care.* SPCK, London.
34 Levenson MR, Jennings PA, Aldwin CM *et al.* (2005) Self-transcendence: conceptualization and measurement. *International Journal of Aging and Human Development.* **60**(2): 127–43.
35 Sermabeikian P (1994) Our clients, ourselves: the spiritual perspective and social work practice. *Social Work.* **39**(2): 178–83.
36 Myco F (1985) The non-believer in the healthcare situation. In: McGilloway O, Myco F (eds) *Nursing and Spiritual Care.* Harper and Row, London.
37 Saunders C (1995) *Living With Dying, A Guide to Palliative Care.* Oxford University Press, Oxford.
38 Murray RB, Zentner JB (1989) *Nursing Concepts for Health Promotion.* Prentice Hall, London.
39 McSherry W (2000) Educational issues surrounding the teaching of spirituality. *Nursing Standard.* **14**(42): 40–3.
40 Bash A (2004) Spirituality: the emperor's new clothes? *Journal of Clinical Nursing.* **13**(1): 11–16.
41 Walter T (1997) The ideology and organization of spiritual care: three approaches. *Palliative Medicine.* **11**: 21–30.
42 Benjamin P, Looby J (1998) Defining the nature of spirituality in the context of Maslow's and Rogers's theories. *Counseling and Values.* **42**: 92–100.
43 Small N (1998) Spirituality and hospice care. In: Cobb M, Robshaw V (eds) *The Spiritual Challenge of Health Care.* Churchill Livingstone, Edinburgh.
44 Markham I (1998) Spirituality and the world faiths. In: Cobb M, Robshaw V (eds) *The Spiritual Challenge of Health Care.* Churchill Livingstone, Edinburgh.
45 Walter T (2002) Spirituality in palliative care: opportunity or burden? *Palliative Medicine.* **16**: 133–9.
46 Chao CC, Chen C, Yen M (2002) The essence of spirituality of terminally ill patients. *Journal of Nursing Research.* **10**(4): 237–44.
47 Narayanasamy A, Gates B, Swinton J (2002) Spirituality and learning disabilities: a qualitative study. *British Journal of Nursing.* **11**(14): 948–57.
48 Fawcett J (1993) *Analysis and Evaluation of Conceptual Models of Nursing.* FA Davies, Philadelphia, PA.
49 Courtenay B (1993) Personhood – personal and faith development. In: Jarvis P, Walters N (eds) *Adult Education and Theological Interpretations.* Krieger, Malabar, Florida.
50 MacKinlay F (2001) *The Spiritual Dimension of Ageing.* Jessica Kingsley, London.
51 Kenny G (1999) The iron cage and the spider's web: children's spirituality and the hospital environment. *Paediatric Nursing.* **11**(5): 20–3.
52 Smith J, McSherry W (2004) Spirituality and child development: a concept analysis. *Journal of Advanced Nursing.* **45**(3): 307–15.
53 Moore J (1980) *Sexuality Spirituality, A Study of Feminine/Masculine Relationship.* Element, Tisbury, Wiltshire.
54 McSherry W, Cash K (2003) The language of spirituality: an emerging taxonomy. *International Journal of Nursing Studies.* **41**: 151–61.
55 Nolan P, Crawford P (1997) Towards a rhetoric of spirituality in mental healthcare. *Journal of Advanced Nursing.* **26**(2): 289–94.
56 Greenstreet W (1996) *Teaching Spirituality in Nursing.* Unpublished MA dissertation, Faculty Education, Canterbury Christ Church University.
57 McSherry W, Watson R (2002) Spirituality in nursing care: evidence of a gap between theory and practice. *Journal of Clinical Nursing.* **11**(6): 843–4.

CHAPTER 2

Past and present discourses

Wendy Greenstreet

Introduction

Discourse represents 'a distinct way of thinking, seeing and conversing about a particular phenomena, all of which create a virtual "arena", ruling some ways of thinking as legitimate and others as not'[1] (p.15). In healthcare, medicine's emergence as a dominant discourse in relation to disease of the body has impacted on the standing of spirituality as an aspect of care. This chapter will consider how the art of care within religious orders was replaced by the science of biomedical treatment as the legitimate means of managing the human experience of illness. This is followed by discussion of holistic care as a modern interpretation of care delivery. Using the art of care to deliver science-based treatment increases the potential of a more comprehensive fulfilment of client/patient need and acknowledges spirituality as a perspective of care. Spirituality, as a term that now figures in social and many professional agendas, is then considered in relation to contemporary views on difference and commonalities of interpretation.

From religious roots to researching the benefits of religion

Religious professionals

Spirituality is often mistakenly equated with religion. This is not surprising given that the roots of the caring professions that predate modernity have evolved from a religious vocation. In nursing, for example, Christianity provided a religion for the 'sick', God in Christ having shared in the suffering of humanity.[2] The emphasis was on spiritual healing and supportive care rather than physical cure.[3] Nurses derived spiritual fulfilment themselves by finding meaning in the care they provided for the sick.[4] Similarly, Culliford[5] describes medicine as once fully bound up with religion.

Some individual, contemporary professionals may still see their practice as a religious vocation and live their faith in the provision of care to those in need. Chan *et al.*[6] reflect the motivation of doctors with different religious faiths choosing to practise medicine. For example, Chan[6] refers to Buddha's teaching centred on how to deal with human suffering and sorrow; Pickering[6] chose medicine as an opportunity to fulfil a Christian need to serve others; and Pai[6] believes that his practice of Hinduism is a way of life and so brings key features such as tolerance and truth to his practice of medicine. Rassool[7] also explains that, for Islamic nurses, there is no spirituality without religious thoughts and practices, and that religion is a way of life. This intrinsic acting out of religious belief may provide altruistic drive to individual professional performance, but it is important to differentiate between practitioner religious fervour and patient/client philosophy to ensure that there is no attempt, either consciously or subconsciously, to proselytise.

Reason and secularisation

However, overall the professional view has undergone a fundamental change from an underpinning religious philosophy to one of utilitarian secularism. Dawson[8] suggests that the gradual split between the art of healing and its spiritual base can be traced to early Greek thinkers whose philosophy lent itself to the examination of the physical rather than the spiritual for causation. However, the 'Age of Reason'[8] (p.285) opened this split into a chasm. The enlightenment of the eighteenth century resulted in the questioning of traditional Christian values. A century later, religious orders were not able to cope with the demands of an increasing population and advances in medical practice.[9] As a consequence, religious vocation was replaced by humanistic philanthropy epitomised in Nightingale's covenantal model of care, being based on mutual sharing and personal commitment[2] that required practitioners of suitable 'character' based on Judeo-Christian moral values rather than religious practice.[10] The analytical ambience of the twentieth century saw a drive for professionalisation and an increasing requirement for evidence-based practice in health and social care professions.[11] The search for evidence has contributed to attempts to measure the impact of religion on the outcomes of care and treatment empirically. This reflects a significant shift from an ethos of religious professions to the professions' secular interest in patient/client religion.

Research and religion

Research studies explore the benefit and burden of religion in a variety of clinical contexts, including rehabilitation,[12] malignancy,[13] mental health[14,15] and end-of-life care.[16] Findings suggest that religion was a source of consolation for some in rehabilitation, that religious coping may help cancer survivors 'block out' the experience of cancer and related complications, and in mental health, religiousness was mildly associated with fewer symptoms of depression but could be either a source of strength or burden to the patient suffering schizophrenia. In facing death, people were often drawn closer to traditional religious beliefs, and communication about religious faith may constitute an important part of final conversations.

There are potentially a number of reasons why those who have a sincere religious faith are likely to experience some health benefits. Mohr and Huguelet[15] outline these succinctly as behavioural, social, psychological and physiological mechanisms (Table 2.1). Hill and Pargament[17] discuss these benefits in more detail (Table 2.2).

Religious belief and practice bring people closer to the transcendent, however that transcendence or 'God' is defined. Hill and Pargament[17] use attachment theory to suggest that experiencing a secure connection with God should be a source of

Table 2.1 Religion's potential link to health[15]

Mechanism	Means
Behavioural	Healthy lifestyle
Social	Religious groups provide supportive communities for their members
Psychological	Beliefs about God, ethics, human relationships, life and death
Physiological	Religious practices elicit a relaxation response

Table 2.2 Potential health benefits of religious faith[17]

Secure connection with 'God'	lower physiological responses to stress
	lower levels of loneliness
Religious coping methods	prayer
	rites of passage
	meditation
Avoidance of vices	gluttony
	lust
	pride
	envy
Practice of virtues	forgiveness
	gratitude
	hope
Social support	source of self-esteem, companionship
	'support convoy' throughout life

strength and lower physiological responses to stress as well as resulting in lower levels of loneliness. Also, religion provides a framework that facilitates access to religious coping methods such as, prayer, rites of passage and meditation. Similarly, religious practice increases the likely avoidance of vices, for example gluttony, lust, envy and pride, and increased efforts to practise virtues such as forgiveness, gratitude and hope which are associated with physical and mental health. Hill and Pargament[17] also outline the health benefits that individuals derive from the support of members, leaders and clergy in their religious congregations. As with other forms of social support, these include a valuable source of self-esteem, information and companionship. However, they also refer to religious systems as providing a 'support convoy' that can accompany the individual throughout their life. The people who make up the convoy may change, but would share a set of values and a world-view, even in very difficult circumstances. Prayers offered on behalf of the individual, and a belief in God working through others, are also offered as further sources of religious support.

However, Hill and Pargament[17] also point out that negative religious coping can disadvantage the maintenance or recovery of health. Religious struggles are traditionally described as pivotal moments that may lead individuals onward to growth and a sense of wellbeing or result in a loss of faith that may undermine health.

Fitchett *et al.*,[12] for example, found that anger with God was predictive of poor recovery of functional ability in those undergoing medical rehabilitation. These struggles are potentially very distressing, eliciting ultimate questions and concerns that challenge sacred core beliefs.[17] Doubts about the trustworthiness of others may stem from conflict with congregation or clergy, and self-worth may be questioned if certainty about God's nature is shaken. Stressful events may be construed as a sign of abandonment or punishment by God.[18]

From the rise of science to the limitation of meta-narrative

The enlightenment and science

The enlightenment resulted in a cultural and intellectual shift in healthcare that saw the rise of the medical sciences.[19] This shift contributed to a twentieth-century meta-narrative that offered a framework to seek answers by breaking things into manageable (controllable) sections characteristic of modernity.[20] Rather than being considered as an integral whole, a person was reduced to constituting parts; the body was seen as a collection of biological systems that lend themselves to measurement and the rigour of empirical study. The consequences of modernity in healthcare saw the replacement of a covenantal model of care by a contractual approach that is focused on a task accomplishment style of delivery and neglects the soul, spirit and numinous. The emphasis is on physical treatment to achieve cure rather than supportive or spiritual care.

More recently, spirituality has achieved recognition in science's quest for causality and has been diagnosed as being neurological. Zohar and Marshall[21] refer to research by a neurobiologist, Persinger, who, knowing of the predisposition of people with temporal epilepsy to have profound spiritual experiences, used electrical stimulation of the temporal lobe of the brain to induce a sense of the divine. Daaleman[22] refers to technological research that has produced similar findings. In this research, single photon emission computed tomographic images of the brains of Buddhists and Franciscan nuns during meditation demonstrated localised neural activity within the brain.

The challenge of existential questions

However, science is limited by boundaries and fails to meet the challenge of existential questions (Giddens 1991, cited[23]) such as those posed by individuals facing loss, suffering and death.[23] Spirituality is similar in one way to science in seeking the answers to questions,[24] but mostly complements science in relying not on objective evidence but on subjective expression in unravelling a phenomenon that is not measurable and is too amorphous to be described adequately by the intellectual use of language.

Medical science's reliance on a meta-narrative that worshipped the 'false god of objectivity'[25] (p.12) for answers to all questions failed to acknowledge that the enlightenment's rejection of narrow Christian values did not wholly reject the idea of 'God'.[26] The growing complexities of science and technology that drive and dominate Western materialism, and an increasing number of Eastern societies, do not answer questions of meaning in life.[27] In the UK, data from the 2001 Census reflects a considerable religious-spiritual feeling in that responses to the question on religion show around 75% of the population associated themselves with a recognised religion and only 16% stated they had no religion.[26] However, this is not reflected in church attendance in England, where there was a reduction of almost 4% attendance between 1979 and 1998 (Brierly 2000b, cited[28]), but might reflect a reinterpretation of the word religion in a society that values individualism. Davie (1994, cited[28]) found that between 66% and 75% of British society wanted to believe but not to participate in religious practice. The humanistic understanding of spirituality is viewed as more basic than traditional expressions of religiousity in being that which concerns itself with the ongoing problems of human existence.[29]

'Alternative' movements drawing on varied religious philosophies provide different means of the search for meaning. MacLaren[26] explains that the New Age movement's roots are in theosophy, and includes Hindu, Buddhist and pagan theories. The movement is also characterised by ecological concerns, which stem largely from the success of science and technology. New Age shifts focus from a collective view of religion to the 'self' that offers a new strength and meaning to individuals. Postmodern individualism is pervasive in Western societies and in its institutions. Consequently, it has resulted in a shift from a paternalistic, benevolent ethos in delivery of professional care to an increased autonomy for, and by, those using health and social care services.

The emergence of 'holistic' philosophy

It is not surprising that one of the greatest challenges to a medical model focused on cure stemmed from its inability to offer guidance on care of the dying. A new model, one of 'holistic', person-centred care that challenged reductionist philosophy, was introduced by Cicely Saunders in the modern hospice movement initiated in the UK in the 1960s. Multiprofessional in her own right, having qualifications in nursing, social work and medicine,[30] she perceived care to be multi-dimensional constituting physical, social, psychological and spiritual perspectives (Figure 2.1).

These aspects of care can also be portrayed as mirrored in the individual patient or client and are better depicted as an integrated 'whole' (*see* Figure 1.1) in which spirituality may constitute a significant part of the 'hidden' self (*see* Figure 1.2). In a postmodern culture, different forms of spirituality fulfil each individual's quest 'to find meaning', or 'to believe', which cannot be amalgamated into a collective 'norm' if they are to remain valuable.

A 'holistic' model of care demands a shift in focus from the efficiency and task of medical treatment to authentic relationships[31] responsive to an individual's needs and reciprocal in nature.[32] The implication then is that the professional is personally able to contribute to care by the very nature of their relationship with those in need of health and social care as well as, or regardless of, any prescribed action to administer treatment.

The way the professional uses 'self' in relation to spirituality as a perspective of care has in itself been a contentious issue. Spirituality as a personal quality of the

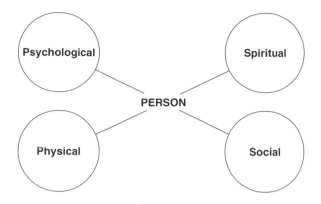

Figure 2.1 Spirituality in the context of multidimensional, person-centred care.

professional carer would influence their beliefs, experiences and practices, and underpin professional activity and the nature of the caring relationship. This does not need to be articulated by the professional but would reflect their intrinsic religiosity. Alternatively, a professional's own spirituality can be a more public quality, articulated in dealings with those in need of their care. This can be problematical in pluralistic health and social care settings. A suggestion by MacLaren[26] for nurses regarding this issue may well be applicable to other health and social care professionals, and that is to be like anthropologists, putting their own beliefs to one side and observe the other's reality without interpretation according to their own ideas. Similarly, Silver[33] exemplifies the contemporary use of secular terminology as more politically expedient; 'the dignity of human life' having replaced the notion of 'the sanctity of the soul' (p.338). In this way, language is inclusive of spiritualities rather than singular religiosity.

Spirituality and regulation

Professionalisation of health and social care has resulted in a proliferation of codes of practice that are public statements of the values and principles of each profession. Regularly updated, these codes reflect each profession's stance on spirituality as a perspective of care. This stance can be implicit, explicit or not acknowledged.

   The Code of Ethics and Professional Conduct for Occupational Therapy in England,[34] for example, makes no explicit statement regarding spiritual care. However, Udell and Chandler[35] believe that spirituality is alluded to in the section outlining the occupational therapist's responsibility to respect and uphold client uniqueness, autonomy and dignity. Howard and Howard[36] explain that one way in which occupational therapists relate occupation to spirituality, as ultimate meaning, is through the use of time. Creative activity provides the means of escaping the binding effects that time has on us. Also, the rhythm of rest and activity in the greater rhythms of life bring balance and health to a person. Therefore the therapist helps people find themselves by losing themselves in occupation. Spirituality in occupational therapy appears, therefore, to be explicit in the profession's philosophy, if not in their code of practice.

Professional codes and guidelines for nurses are more explicit. The Nursing and Midwifery Council's Code of Professional Conduct[37] holds registered nurses, midwives and health visitors personally accountable for ensuring that 'the interests and dignity of patients and clients, irrespective of gender, age, race, ability, sexuality, economic status, lifestyle, culture and religious or political beliefs' (p.4) are promoted and respected. Similarly, the International Council of Nurse's Code of Ethics[38] requires nurses to promote an environment that respects the values, customs and spiritual beliefs of those in their care and their significant others. Also, the significance of nursing assessment of spiritual need and delivery of spiritual care is made explicit as part of the provision of holistic care as a standard for entry to the professional register.[39]

The College of Radiographers' Statements of Professional Conduct[40] does not permit radiographers 'to be selective' (p.11) in their duty of care on the grounds of religion, but otherwise makes no statement that links to spiritual care. The Code of Practice for Social Care Workers[41] takes a firmer stance in requiring practitioners to treat each person as an individual, 'respecting diversity and different cultures and values' (1.1, 1.6).

Socio-political recognition of spirituality in healthcare is reflected in The Patient's Charter,[42] requiring staff to respect patients' religious, spiritual and cultural needs at all times. More recently the Department of Health has produced guidelines for spiritual care.[43] An increase in public statement(s) by either professional or government institutions regarding the spiritual aspect of care potentiates its acknowledgement and provision in health and social care contexts.

Polarisation or conflation as contemporary views of spirituality

Tripartite tension

Spirituality is used as a secular, sacred or religious term. The tension between the use of these terms hinges on whether they are seen as reflecting absolute phenomena in their own right or whether they are extractions of an overriding complex but single phenomenon. Unruh et al.[44] suggest that, regardless of whether a secular, sacred or religious definition of spirituality is preferred, they are all associated with a search for answers to the same fundamental questions (Box 2.1). What differs is the framework in which the answers to the questions are constructed.

Box 2.1 Fundamental questions[44]

- How was the world created?
- What is the origin of life?
- Is there life after death?
- How do we account for the presence of good and evil in the world?
- What are our obligations to each other and the world around us?
- Is there redemption or forgiveness for wrongs and omissions?
- What is the meaning and purpose of human life?
- Why do bad things happen to good people?

Religions have a theistic doctrine that provides answers or teachings as a response to these fundamental questions. Unruh *et al.*[44] describe a sacred approach as one that may reject aspects of a theistic framework but retain a belief in a higher being or ultimate truth that may guide the search for answers to spiritual questions. A secular approach rejects theistic and sacred frameworks and seeks alternative sources of guidance, such as humanistic or existential philosophy.

Whitehead[45] supports polarisation of the metaphysical and existential views of spirituality. He claims defining existential health to be a less elusive task than defining spirituality, which is 'too pluralistic and eclectic' for definitional development (p.681). Metaphysical health is described as centred on the individual's belief in the presence of a deity/god/supernatural being that is an external resource, whereas existential health manifests itself within the 'emotional mind' (p.680), as an inner resource. However, this polarisation fails to reflect the dynamic personal element of belief, and increasingly reflects only the personal, subjective experience of secular spirituality.[17] Therefore polarisation limits care to the intellectually definable rather than the need of human experience.

Cultural stereotyping

Polarisation of the cultural variables of individualism and collectivism, typically presumed to reflect Western and Eastern experiences and behaviours respectively, result in assumptions and stereotyping. Eastern and Western religions are therefore compared, for example by seeking in Christianity the sources of Western individualism or in Taoism and Buddhism the sources of Eastern collectivism.[46] Individualism is associated with a bounded, independent self/person separate from the 'other' in relationship. Collectivism is associated with an interdependent relationship and ill-defined boundaries between the self/person and 'others'.[46] Individualistic cultures value open and direct communication, and collectivistic cultures are contrasted as passive and reserved.[47] In considering mental health in Asian women, Wong and Tsang[47] illustrate the error of such assumptions and stereotyping. The ways in which these women perceived spirituality were as varied as those described in Western literature, for example:

- **Religious**: 'But perhaps because you experience a blow in your life, you begin to think about how the principles of life unfold, why I encounter so many difficulties, why bad things happen to me. You would begin to think about the reasons and want to study what being human is all about, what life is all about. Religion gives many answers. There are many different paths: Catholicism, Christianity, Buddhism, they have different approaches. Because you have come to the time when [religion] speaks to your need, it becomes easier for you to become more humble to acknowledge an external power beyond you' (Taiwanese, p.460).
- **Extrinsic religiosity**: 'That Korean community has a lot of Christians is not necessarily because their faith in God is so strong and they are so religious. You should not think like that – It is a kind of social network – Because you feel lonely here, it'd better to go to church and meet people and get any information' (Korean, p.463).
- **Secular**: 'My picture is like, you see, there are music, flowers, leaves, animals especially a cat, which is my favourite pet; and smile and a heart. The heart is in

the heart shape of love. This kind of love is with everyone and for everyone; not for your family only but for everyone that you have connection with. That is of spiritual significance to me. It is the situation, whether you are working or playing, entertaining, where there is always the harmony, which uses love to treat each other' (Vietnamese, p.461).

These examples demonstrate the need for professional carers to explore individual experiences and behaviours of clients/patients rather than expect stereotypical responses associated with polarisation of cultural variables.

'The between'

Sampson[46] challenges the polarisation of the person–other relationship as either being individualistically independent or collectively interdependent. Rather than independent relationships characteristic of individualism, which see others as separate, as instruments of service, as models, helpers or opponents, he advocates desirable relationships as not being concerned with boundaries but formative dialogue; 'one cannot truly be a person apart from being in dialogue with others; others therefore are central to the very existence and possibility of being an individual in the first place' (p.1429). Also, in contrast to independent relationships, in which the person remains the star and the 'other' is an audience that is watching, commenting or applauding, in formative dialogue, person and 'other' are equal partners in a process of mutual formation; 'in a genuine dialogue [a] person is responsive to the particularity of the other, to the other's uniqueness and otherness' (p.1430) and 'That which is most fundamental about the person is not to be discovered either within any individual person or in the collectivity but exists in what Buber (1965) referred to as the third sphere, "the between"' (p.1429). This conflation of individualism and collectivism has potentially much to offer health and social care professionals in understanding where and how the fundamental spirituality of a person may be located.

Analogy and meaning

Rather than polarise the different interpretation of meanings of spirituality, van Leeuwen and Cusveller[48] refer to a 'family of different yet connected meanings' (p.237). Similarly, McSherry and Cash[49] outline a taxonomy of descriptors that are identified within the definitions of spirituality, which range from the religious to the existential and mystical (Table 2.3).

Conflation of a mixture of the components of the taxonomy, of varying strengths and flavours according to an individual's world-view or religious belief, in a 'cocktail' of spirituality is an analogy that works well in conveying the concept as fluid, particularly in relation to lifespan development, illness or emotional stress. The sequencing and priorities of descriptors change from one individual to the next. This taxonomy is inclusive of the religious, sacred and secular views of spirituality.

Table 2.3   Descriptors in a taxonomy of spirituality[49]

Theistic	belief in supreme being
Religious	belief in a God
Language	'inner strength', 'inner peace'
Cultural, political, social ideologies	ideology influences attitudes, behaviours
Phenomenological	life is learnt from experience
Existential	being, finding meaning and purpose
Quality of life	implicit in definitions of spirituality
Mystical	relationship with transcendent

Conclusion

Historically, religious individuals contributed to health and social welfare by offering healing and support. Some contemporary health and social care professionals find spiritual fulfilment in their faith in, and practise of, a religion, but this is not a requirement of providing spiritual care and should not be imposed on those requiring the services of professional carers. In an increasingly secular society, where utilitarian interest is in the outcomes of health and social care, professionals, rather than necessarily being religious, research into the value of religion in clients/patients who use their faith and the practice of ritual as a source of coping. Professionalisation has seen the spiritual dimension of care neglected and a reliance on medical science focused on cure.

However, science and technology do not have answers to questions about the meaning of life. When life itself is challenged by illness, hardship and dying that science cannot cure, a 'holistic' approach to care that includes the spiritual dimension and acknowledges client/patient choice facilitates healing. The term 'spirituality' is polysemic in having different meanings. This is evident in a temporal sense in its past and current use, in its cultural interpretation and in the use of comparative analogy that implies mix and fluidity. It is not in the difference that the greatest strength of the concept lies but in 'the between', in understanding the relationship in which spirituality is located

References

1   Barry A, Yuill C (2002) *Understanding Health, A Sociological Introduction.* Sage, London.
2   Bradshaw A (1994) *Lighting the Lamp, The Spiritual Dimension of Nursing Care.* Scutari Press, Harrow.
3   Greenstreet W (1999) Teaching spirituality in nursing: a literature review. *Nurse Education Today.* **19**: 649–58.
4   Narayanasamy A (1999) Learning spiritual dimensions of care from a historical perspective. *Nurse Education Today.* **19**: 386–95.
5   Culliford L (2002) Spirituality and clinical care: spiritual values and skills are increasingly recognised as necessary aspects of clinical care. *BMJ.* **325**(7378): 1434–5.
6   Chan K, Pickering M, Pai S *et al.* (2003) Doctors and their faiths. *BMJ Career Focus.* **326**: 135.

7 Rassool GH (2000) The Crescent and Islam: healing, nursing and the spiritual dimension. Some considerations towards an understanding of the Islamic perspectives on caring. *Journal of Advanced Nursing.* **32**(6): 1476–84.

8 Dawson PJ (1997) A reply to Goddard's 'spirituality as integrative energy'. *Journal of Advanced Nursing.* **25**(2): 282–9.

9 Baly ME (1980) *Nursing and Social Change.* Heinemann, London.

10 Widerquist JG (1992) The spirituality of Florence Nightingale. *Nursing Research.* **41**(1): 49–55.

11 Le May A (1999) *Evidence-based Practice.* NT Books, London.

12 Fitchett G, Rybarczyk B, DeMarco G *et al.* (1999) The role of religion in medical rehabilitation outcomes: a longitudinal study. *American Psychological Association.* **44**(4): 333–53.

13 Gall TL (2004) The role of religious coping in adjustment to prostate cancer. *Cancer Nursing.* **27**(6): 454–61.

14 Smith T, McCullough M, Poll J (2003) Religiousness and depression: evidence for a main effect and moderating influence of stressful life events. *American Psychological Association.* **129**(4): 614–36.

15 Mohr S, Huguelet P (2004) The relationship between schizophrenia and religion and its implications for care. *Swiss Med Wkly.* **134**: 369–76.

16 Keeley MP (2004) Final conversations: survivors' memorable messages concerning religious faith and spirituality. *Health Communication.* **16**(1): 87–104.

17 Hill P, Pargament K (2003) Advances in the conceptualisation and measurement of religion and spirituality: implications for physical and mental health research. *American Psychological Association.* **58**(1): 64–74.

18 Pargament KI (1997) *The Psychology of Religion and Coping: theory, research practice.* Guilford Press, New York.

19 Kroeker PT (1997) Spirituality and occupational therapy in a secular culture. *Canadian Journal of Occupational Therapy.* **64**(3): 122–6.

20 Small N (2001) Theories of grief: a critical review. In: Hockey J, Katz J, Small N (eds) *Grief, Mourning and Death Ritual.* Open University Press, Buckingham.

21 Zohar D, Marshall I (2000) *Spiritual Intelligence, the Ultimate Intelligence.* Bloomsbury, London.

22 Daaleman TP (2004) Religion, spirituality, and the practice of medicine. *The Journal of the American Board of Family Practice.* **17**(5): 370–6.

23 Hennery N (2003) Constructions of spirituality in contemporary nursing theory. *Journal of Advanced Nursing.* **42**(6): 550–7.

24 McSherry W, Draper P (1998) The debates emerging from the literature surrounding the concept of spirituality as applied to nursing. *Journal of Advanced Nursing.* **27**(4): 683–91.

25 Fish D (1998) *Appreciating Practice in the Caring Professions: refocusing professional development and practitioner research.* Butterworth Heinemann, Oxford.

26 MacLaren J (2004) A kaleidoscope of understandings: spiritual nursing in a multi-faith society. *Journal of Advanced Nursing.* **45**(5): 457–62.

27 Jarvis P (1993) Meaning, being and learning. In: Jarvis P, Walters N (eds) *Adult Education and Theological Interpretations.* Krieger, Malabar, Florida.

28 Furman LD, Benson PW, Grimwood C *et al.* (2004) Religion and spirituality in social work education and direct practice at the millennium: a survey of UK social workers. *British Journal of Social Work.* **34**: 767–92.

29 Elkins DN, Hedstrom LJ, Hughes LL *et al.* (1988) Toward a humanistic-phenomenological spirituality. *Journal of Humanistic Psychology.* **28**(4): 5–18.

30 Hockley J (1997) The evolution of the hospice approach. In: Clark D, Hockley J, Ahmedzai S (eds) *New Themes in Palliative Care.* Open University Press, Buckingham.

31 Aranda S (2001) Silent voices, hidden practices: exploring undiscovered aspects of cancer nursing. *International Journal of Palliative Nursing.* **7**(4): 178–85.

32 Aranda S, Street A (1999) Being authentic and being a chameleon: nurse-patient interaction revisited *Nursing Inquiry.* **6**: 75–82.

33 Silver LM (2003) Biotechnology and conceptualisations of the soul. *Cambridge Quarterly of Health Care Ethics.* **12**: 335–41.

34   College of Occupational Therapists (2000) *The Code of Ethics and Professional Conduct for Occupational Therapists.* College of Occupational Therapists, London.

35   Udell L, Chandler C (2000) The role of the occupational therapist in addressing the spiritual needs of clients. *British Journal of Occupational Therapy.* **63**(10): 489–94

36   Howard BS, Howard JR (1996) Occupation as spiritual activity. *The American Journal of Occupational Therapy.* **51**(3): 181–5.

37   Nursing and Midwifery Council (2002) *Code of Professional Conduct.* NMC, London.

38   International Council of Nurses (2000) *The International Council Code of Ethics.* ICN, Geneva.

39   Nursing and Midwifery Council (2004) *Standards of Proficiency for Preregistration Nursing Education.* NMC, London.

40   The College of Radiographers (2004) *Statements of Professional Conduct.* College of Radiographers, London.

41   General Social Care Council (2004) *Codes of Practice.* General Social Care Council, London.

42   Department of Health (2001) *The Patient's Charter.* DoH, London.

43   Department of Health (2003) *NHS Chaplaincy: meeting the religious and spiritual needs of patients and staff.* DoH, London.

44   Unruh AM, Versnel J, Kerr N (2002) Spirituality unplugged: a review of commonalities and contentions, and a resolution. *Canadian Journal of Occupational Therapy.* **February**: 5–19.

45   Whitehead D (2003) Beyond the metaphysical: health-promoting existential mechanisms and their impact on the health status of clients. *Journal of Clinical Nursing.* **12**(5): 678–88.

46   Sampson E (2000) Reinterpreting individualism and collectivism: their religious roots and monologic versus dialogic person-other relationship. *American Psychologist.* **55**(12): 1425–32.

47   Wong YR, Tsang AK (2004) When Asian immigrant women speak: from mental health to strategies of being. *American Journal of Orthopsychiatry.* **74**(4): 456–66.

48   van Leeuwen R, Cusveller B (2004) Nursing competencies for spiritual care. *Journal of Advanced Nursing.* **48**(3): 234–46.

49   McSherry W, Cash K (2003) The language of spirituality: an emerging taxonomy. *International Journal of Nursing Studies.* **41**: 151–61.

CHAPTER 3

Spiritual wellbeing and spiritual distress

Wendy Greenstreet

Introduction

Spirituality can be depicted as a continuum of spiritual need from spiritual wellbeing and its association with health at one extreme, and spiritual distress associated with despair at the other.[1] In this way, spiritual wellbeing is a continuous variable that Whitehead[2] believes to be not so much an issue of whether or not we have it, but more a question of how much? As every person has a spiritual dimension, so everyone has spiritual needs, although such needs are not always recognised even by the individual. Spiritual health reflects fulfilled needs, and spiritual despair a significant deficit. Between the two extremes there is potentially a wide range of levels of unfulfilled spiritual need. This chapter will explore what is meant by spiritual wellbeing and then consider spiritual intelligence as a means of achieving and maintaining spiritual health. Similarly, the meaning of spiritual need and spiritual distress will be examined. Some thought will then be given to assessing the spiritual needs of those receiving care in health and social care settings, whether this is possible, and if so, when and how this can be achieved.

Spiritual wellbeing

Spiritual wellbeing is usually described by its cause and effect. Recorded history and philosophers associate happiness as a source of wellbeing.[3] The construct of happiness exists across cultures, but aspects of life that constitute happiness are weighted differently in different cultures.[4] The effect of spiritual wellbeing is characterised by serenity, courage and wisdom.[5] It is an indication of a person's quality of life in the spiritual dimension or simply an indication of their spiritual health.[6] In health and social care, clients/patients may make statements implying spiritual health, for example:

- I feel that life is a positive experience
- my relationship with God helps me not to feel lonely
- I believe there is some real purpose for my life.[7]

Booth[8] describes healthy spirituality as being a power within us that enables us to make choices and take responsibility for our lives. Thus responsibility is a response-*ability*, meaning the ability to respond. Healthy spirituality is not only found in acts of kindness and self-sacrifice, but also in setting boundaries, in saying 'no'. Booth goes on to explain that we are most spiritually healthy when we allow ourselves to be real, and so less than perfect. He illustrates this by the following:

> As the Skin Horse says in *The Velveteen Rabbit*, the process of becoming real is a lengthy one; it doesn't happen all at once. 'You BECOME. That's why it doesn't happen to people who break easily or have sharp edges, or who have to be carefully kept. Generally, by the time you are REAL, most of your hair has been loved off, and your eyes drop out and you get loose in the joints and very shabby. But these things don't matter at all, because once you are REAL, you can't be ugly, except to people who don't understand'.[9] (pp.12–13)

Diener *et al.*[4] review the progress achieved in three decades of research concerning subjective wellbeing, which is the measure of individuals' perceived happiness.[10] Findings link affective styles and the potential genetic influence of brain hormones and receptor sites to wellbeing. Similarly, healthy spirituality has been linked to the emotional self,[8] and spirituality has been found to have a neurological location within the brain.[11]

Diener *et al.*[4] refer to the cultural influence of individualism and collectivism on self-esteem in relation to wellbeing, the former utilising strategies to maintain personal self-esteem and the latter valuing the group above the individual. Friedemann *et al.*[12] also link culture to spiritual health. They describe health as achieving congruence, a balance between control and spirituality. The tension created by incongruence results in anxiety, and individuals buffer the effect of this tension by striving to regain a more harmonious balance. The emphasis in balance on either control or spirituality is individual and dependent on culture, beliefs and values.

In a culture that supports individualism, control is highly valued. Control is considered a means of protection from inherent vulnerability and provides a sense of security. Therefore, to control threatening change, such as serious illness and associated anxiety, individuals struggle to re-establish pre-existing conditions as far as possible by planning and deliberate behavioural strategies involving seeking information, medication and technological application as a means of achieving this. This struggle for control is individual, familial and societal. Control is not always possible and the incongruence that results may lead to feelings of hopelessness associated with despair and potential spiritual distress.

Human spirituality offers a second means of reducing tension caused by anxiety and so allows a return to a more healthy congruence. It involves intellectual and emotional activity to achieve transcendence of artificial limits. In transcending their immediate situation, individuals are able to sharpen their perception of our dependence on a wider universal order that we are unable to control. Spirituality in this sense is liberating and allows health to be possible in the presence of disease. Friedemann *et al.*[12] give the example of the process of organ failure as a natural occurrence in older people, which as such, is congruent with a universal order and, therefore, the disease process may not contradict health. Similarly, a situation in which a person accepts mortality without becoming excessively anxious is one where spirituality has allowed the experience of health. However, where patients struggle to gain control by continuing invasive treatment that is futile in the face of the universal order, an over-reliance on control can result in anxiety, anger and resentment that destroys interpersonal relationships and exacerbates incongruence rather than health.

Spiritual wellness includes setting goals as part of striving for growth.[13] A commitment to goals provides a sense of personal agency and a sense of structure and meaning in life.[4] Aspirations that are realistic and congruent with an individual's personal resources are more likely to enhance wellbeing[14] in that they are achievable. So, in health and social care, spiritual health can be enhanced by client/patient involvement in setting goals for their care that are meaningful to them. Goals are, therefore, the client/patient goals and not prescribed by professional carers. However, professional carers may need to help those in their care understand what is realistic within individual circumstances.

Research supports Booth's[8] view that becoming 'real' is a lengthy process and one associated with increasing age. Diener *et al.*[4] found studies demonstrating that older adults had a closer fit between their ideal self and actual self-perceptions and that this impacted goal setting in adversity. Rather than assimilative coping strategies that required changing life circumstances to personal preferences, there was an increasing tendency to use accommodative coping with ageing that required adjusting personal preferences and goals to given situational constraints. Although the link between objective conditions and wellbeing is said to be mediated by expectation,[4] this may also be taken to reflect accepting ageing as a natural process in the universal order. Accommodative coping, therefore, can be taken as a sign of spiritual health in older people. This may explain why research consistently demonstrates the positive association of spiritual wellbeing with coping. Fehring *et al.*[6] give examples of the spiritually well suffering less loneliness as a consequence of arthritic disease, of having vigour despite chronic pulmonary disease and hope regardless of HIV/AIDS.

As an internal coping force, spiritual wellbeing is derived from maximising spiritual drive. This is described as having two dimensions. One is of transcendence in relation to a higher power or God, and represents an individual's ultimate concern, such as life's purpose. The other is an existential transcendent link with others and the environment that determines purpose and satisfaction in life.[15] Landis[15] suggests that interaction between these two spiritual dimensions is continuous. However, those who profess secular spirituality are likely to be driven solely by the latter. In either case, spiritual wellbeing is considered an essential internal resource necessary for growth in periods of stress.[15]

Daaleman *et al.*'s[16] study explored patient perceptions of spiritual wellbeing. Participants had prior experience of healthcare with or without chronic illness. Life scheme and positive intentionality were the primary components of the process of events described by patients. Life scheme includes the activity of finding meaning in life and a sense of coherence. Implicit meaning is subsumed in the activity of gathering and processing relevant information, and found meaning, or meaningfulness, is interpretation and understanding of data and events within life's larger context. Positive intentionality is linked to a belief in personal capacity to resource what is needed to achieve goals. They concluded that, for patients, a meaningful life scheme and a high degree of positive intentionality promoted personal agency as the link between health-related spirituality and subjective wellbeing.

Spiritual intelligence

Zohar and Marshall[11] describe spiritual health as a condition of centred wholeness. Spiritual intelligence, or spiritual quotient (SQ) (Table 3.1), provides the means of achieving and maintaining this wholeness.

Table 3.1   Summary of Zohar's SQ advice[17]

Be flexible	a person can swap paradigms only with flexibility
Be self-aware	live with some space and silence
Be holistic	see the big picture
Have a vision	be led by your values
Be open to adversity	learn from death and failure
Stand out against the crowd	be a Good Samaritan
Be open to diversity	reframe – step back
Advance to the edge	being a little uncomfortable is where learning and innovation are most likely to occur

Diener *et al.*'s[4] review of research identified personality as significant in subjective wellbeing. Similarly, Zohar and Marshall[11] identify six patterns or paths leading to greater spiritual intelligence (Table 3.2) from six personality types.

Table 3.2   Six paths leading to greater spiritual intelligence[11]

Duty	belonging
Nurturing	loving, nurturing, protecting
Knowledge	understanding, quest for truth
Personal transformation	creative artistic power
Brotherhood	pursuit of justice
Servant leadership	makes what is felt impossible happen

They suggest that most people will find something relevant to themselves and raising their SQ in more than one path; most will, however, probably find they have one main path. Throughout the lifespan a person's main spiritual path frequently changes either gradually or abruptly due, for example, to mid-life crisis or a traumatic episode. The six basic spiritual paths are offered as a rich 'toolbox' (p.228) of options to solve life's problems.

The first path is the path of duty and is about belonging, co-operating with, contributing to and being nurtured by the community. To walk this path in a spiritually intelligent way it is important to *want* to belong to the group, to make an inner commitment to it, a choice to belong and understand why. Recognising what the codes and myths of the community are and how these are represented symbolically makes the choice one that is beyond conformity. The spiritually intelligent *feel* loyalty to the group, *serve* its interests, *honour* its codes; they *love* the group. The deepest and most sacred path of duty takes those who chose this path beyond the confines of the group, its myth and practices, to a place from which the SQ of the finite group can be put in perspective. From this level the group can be seen as just one of many valid groups.

The second path is that of nurturing and is about loving, nurturing, protecting and making fertile. Spiritual intelligence on this path means being open to others with whom we are in a caring relationship. This requires being receptive and listening to ourselves, risking self-disclosure and being spontaneous. Zohar and Marshall[11] (p.238) cite Rogers (1961) as summing up this path's essential qualities:

> How can I provide a relationship which this person may use for his own personal growth? No approach which relies upon knowledge, upon training, upon the acceptance of something that is *taught*, is of any use. The more that I can be genuine in the relationship, the more helpful it will be. It is only by providing the genuine reality which is in me, that the other person can successfully seek for the reality in him... The relationship is significant to the extent that I feel a continuing desire to understand ... There is also a complete freedom from any type of moral or diagnostic evaluation.

Deep spirituality is described as being about potential; about what we might become or what we are despite what we express, and is not dissimilar to Booth's[8] view of becoming real. This is also true of the 'other' in the relationship. Spiritually intelligent love is transformative, allowing us a higher expression of self and the other to reach beyond themselves.

The third path is the path of knowledge. This ranges from understanding practical problems, through philosophical quest for truth to knowledge of, and ultimate union with, God. This quest, ranging from curiosity to the limits of understanding, is a search for a truer reality beneath appearances. Spiritually intelligent problem solving places the issue in a wider perspective from which it can be seen more clearly and is similar to Friedemann *et al.*'s[12] view of spirituality's contribution to health as well as definitions of transcendence.[18] Reflection on the meaning and value that drives the situation or problem leads on to reflection on alternatives, outcomes and whether the situation can be improved. Zohar and Marshall[11] warn that new knowledge places what we have known in a different light and may invalidate it. Deep knowledge transforms our very being and takes us through 'trial by fire', which may consume who we previously were. For this reason, the path of knowledge is disciplined requiring, study, reflection, meditation and prayer.

The fourth path is one of personal transformation bringing into being the creative artistic power that each of us has to some extent by virtue of being human. The first task on this path is crucial to us all in exploring the heights and depths of ourselves and welding the disparate, fragmented parts into an independent, whole person. Zohar and Marshall[11] give adolescence and middle age as examples of periods when this is a particular need. However, transpersonal integration draws from a deeper level of the self and is most closely associated with personalities who are open to mystical experiences, to more extreme emotions, eccentricity and battle for and potential loss of their sanity. The artistic are particularly conflict-ridden and know and experience extremes, for example elation and despair. Spiritual intelligence is the willingness to face and attempt to resolve conflict, to remember and reflect on dreams, and to engage in creative dialogue with self or others.

The fifth path is the path of brotherhood associated with an apparent unexciting and unexcitable realistic personality type. Zohar and Marshall[11] describe this as possibly one of the most advanced paths to walk in life. The spiritual task of this path is contact with the deeper realm of men achieved by the fearless and uncompromising pursuit of justice. Justice requires a sense of the equality of claims on a person, recognition that people are different and that conflict is part of life. It also sees that everyone has their claim; brotherhood is about the value of all men. This is tested in confronting our feelings for our adversaries. This can lead to a deep respect for opinions that are different from our own, but also for those who hold them.

The sixth and final path is one of servant leadership. This form of leadership makes what is felt impossible happen, creates new ways for people to relate to one another, new ways for businesses to serve society and new ways for society to *be*. Zohar and Marshall[11] give Gandhi, Martin Luther King, Nelson Mandela and the Dalai Lama as recent and contemporary examples. In being the highest of the spiritual paths, it mirrors the heights of Fowler's[19] sixth stage of faith calling for great integrity. Like Fowler's sixth stage, it is associated with a submission to the highest power imaginable. Submission is a challenge for enterprising personality types who wield power, but it is made possible as an act of grace.

Health and social care professionals who have some knowledge of these paths of spiritual intelligence might be better able to understand spiritual diversity in their clients/patients. They might also benefit from reflecting on their awareness of their own spiritual intelligence, its impact on their ability to care for others and their own ability to *be*.

Spiritual need

Fundamentally, spiritual need is about seeking and finding meaning, transcending hardship and suffering.[20] This is supported in published literature where common themes of meaning and transcendence are demonstrated along with the need for relationships that fulfil the need to give and receive love, and the need for hope and personal forgiveness.[1]

Kellehear[20] describes a multidimensional framework of spiritual need that includes the religious, sacred and secular perspectives (Figure 3.1).

The first of three dimensions included in this model is situational and concerns the need to transcend the immediacy of the situation of illness or social hardship. Kellehear suggests that physical symptoms, the loss of the familiarity of work and home environments, together with the alien ambience of healthcare settings may trigger questioning and reflection that attempts to discern purpose, and find hope, meaning and connectedness in these experiences. The second dimension concerns the moral meanings that stem from the immediacy of a person's biographical situation. Examples given are past grief and grievances, dealing with feelings of abandonment, vulnerability or isolation, and possible desire for resolution of past and present dilemmas, as well as opportunities for prayer and forgiveness. The third dimension is religious, and arises out of the immediacy of the cultural situation and the individual's socialisation or current practices. There may be an attempt to seek religious reconciliation, divine forgiveness and opportunities for religious rites, visits by clergy or reading religious literature.

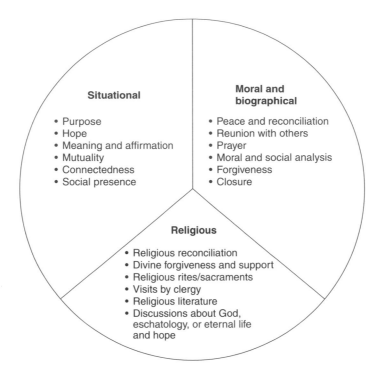

Figure 3.1 Dimensions of spiritual need.[20] Reprinted with permisson. © 2000 Edward Arnold (Publishers) Ltd. *Palliative Medicine.* **14**(2): 153.

Kellehear[20] describes this model in relation to a palliative care context, but it has much to offer health and social care professionals in other settings. The model does not polarise spiritual need as either secular or religious and is flexible in acknowledging spirituality as eclectic and individualistic;[21] a person's needs might be focused primarily in one of the three dimensions, but they may well have additional needs in the other two dimensions. It also demonstrates an overlap in need between the non-religious and religious; prayer, for example, is not exclusively practised by the religious.[22]

Different disease trajectories appear to lead to different patterns of spiritual needs. Murray *et al.*,[21] for example, found that the spiritual needs of patients with lung cancer and their carers were characterised by despair associated with dying, interspersed with periods of hope when they felt better. However, for patients with heart disease and their carers spiritual needs were characterised by hopelessness, isolation and altered self-image relating to chronic illness and disability.

Spiritual distress

Spiritual distress occurs 'when the meaning, value and relationships that secure authentic humanity are seriously threatened'[23] (p.140). Meaninglessness that results in spiritual distress can be mistaken for a symptom of clinical depression but is not responsive to antidepressant medication.[21] O'Brien[24] identifies several components that constitute spiritual distress (Box 3.1).

Box 3.1   Spiritual distress[24]

- Spiritual pain
- Spiritual alienation
- Spiritual anger
- Spiritual anxiety
- Spiritual guilt
- Spiritual loss
- Spiritual despair

O'Brien's[24] definition of spiritual pain is summarised as a deep sense of hurt due to the loss, or separation from, the individual's source of spiritual support, whether a transcendent 'God' or a significant other, such as a life partner.[1] The materialistic concerns of contemporary society can overwhelm an individual's spirit[24] and leave a spiritual void,[25] resulting in spiritual alienation. Spiritual anger, seen in individuals demanding to know 'why?', can result in them blaming their source of spiritual support for the situation they find themselves in. Spiritual anxiety due to fear of loss of spiritual support might manifest itself in unresolved feelings about death and what is beyond it.[26] Spiritual guilt, loss and despair may signal a failure in traversing one's spiritual path, the patient has somehow lost the way.[27] A sense of inadequacy or sinfulness, self-blame and loss of hope would be characteristic of these concepts. Loss of hope may delay patient recovery or even contribute to a premature death, so appropriate support is important.

Hood Morris[28] warns against assuming symptoms of spiritual distress are always unhealthy. She points out that crisis situations that provoke reflection on purpose, personal limitations, the meaning of suffering and issues of control may stimulate development of spiritual qualities. Therefore, depending on the circumstances, spiritual distress may either inhibit spiritual wellbeing or promote spiritual growth.

Assessment of spiritual need

Personal spiritual awareness

All care needs to stem from assessment of patient/client need. Prior to embarking on spiritual assessment of others, health and social care professionals need to consider their own spiritual beliefs, values and biases. An increased spiritual awareness is important to ensure professional carers are able to differentiate between their own spiritual issues and those of the patient/client. In this way, they are more able to remain patient/client-centred and non-judgemental.[29] In caring for the vulnerable, carers need to be aware of their own vulnerability to avoid projecting their own needs and pain into a patient's or client's experience or circumstances. So, spiritual awareness should enhance practitioner confidence in 'staying with'[30] (p.13) those who have spiritual need(s). Exploring personal spirituality and exposure to spiritual experiences tends to increase sensitivity to spiritual need in others.[31] Professionals do not need to deny their own philosophical and spiritual beliefs, but they need to acknowledge their effects.[32] Patients' and clients' spirituality may be challenged by ill health or adversity and professionals need to be sure that they do not intentionally or inadvertently proselytise.

Dossey[33] proposes using reflective questions as a potential means of increasing awareness of personal spirituality. She lists a comprehensive set of questions that are grouped into three sections. The first of these includes questions that assess personal ability to seek meaning and fulfilment in life, experience hope, and accept ambiguity and uncertainty. The second section explores inner strengths and includes questions that assess personal ability to manifest joy, discern strengths, choices, goals and faith. The last section is concerned with relationships with self, others and the transcendent. Questions assess personal positive self-concept, self-esteem and sense of self, capacity to pursue interests, ability to love and forgive self as well as assess personal sense of belonging in the world with 'other'. This questionnaire provides an example of a tool that can assist professionals in exploring and developing self-knowledge that is an important precursor for spiritual assessment and care.[34] It is important for spirituality to be part of health and social care professionals' world-view if this perspective of the patient's care is not to be missed.[35]

Assessment

Spiritual needs change with time and circumstance, and therefore it is not surprising that government guidelines suggest that spiritual issues should be assessed regularly.[36] However, spiritual assessment is not without controversy. Pierpont,[37] for example, points out that there is a difference between gathering information concerning a patient's spirituality and justifying a 'spiritual assessment' (p.562). He believes that those who understand what spirituality is can obtain much information about the spiritual beliefs and practices of patient/client indirectly, by listening to their stories, and that conducting a 'spiritual assessment' may reflect the interest of the professional rather than that of the patient/client. Similarly, Narayanasamy et al.[38] refer to published work that suggests spiritual needs are discerned over time, through ongoing contact and by observation of use of spiritual or religious literature or artefacts, and that many patients/clients feel uncomfortable discussing their beliefs within a structured assessment.

As spirituality is generally focused on its tangible expression through relationships,[39] it is within an established rapport in which the professional is able to be fully 'present' with the client/patient, actively listening[40] and picking up relevant cues, that true spiritual assessment takes place. This form of assessment draws on intuitive and tacit knowledge associated with experience, and is spontaneous in that it is driven by patient/client intimation 'hidden from view' in 'quiet conversations'[41] (p.2) rather than prescriptively determined by the professional. Such intimations often come in the throes of therapy, treatment or care when the professional has sought out the client/patient to fulfil or 'do' some activity for or with them. It is the nature of 'doing' that determines whether activity is delivered within a relationship that is covenantal or contractual, the former facilitating intimations by the patient/client of matters of spirituality providing cues for the professional to consider assessment of need, and the latter promoting an ambience of 'business' focused on task that leaves little room for such moments.

The contractual nature of contemporary health and social care services is not without altruistic intent. McSherry and Ross[42] refer to clinical governance and evidence-based practice driving the desire to quantify and measure care to raise standards and reduce risk. However, clinical audit requires records of practice and a given standard to measure the quality of that practice against. Prescribed assessment 'tools' raise the profile of aspects of care in requiring tasks to be performed that result in a recorded activity and provide data for audit trails. Spirituality does not lend itself to standardisation, and using a tool to assess and record spiritual need often results in using 'the language of rationality that speaks of the normal and the pathological, of processes and systems'[43] (p.105) that cannot convey the more personal message of emotional and spiritual need of or for care.

Assessment tools

Consideration of tools to assess spiritual needs must start with clarifying what they are able to measure. Bash[44] explains that spiritual experience is not capable of being scientifically measured. However, tools can help professionals to describe and identify the outward expression of spiritual experience, the views, feelings and behaviours that may result. The sources of tools available to assess spiritual aspects of wellbeing or spiritual need appear to fall into three categories. These are measurement tools specifically for research purposes, those found in published literature and the unpublished, developed in practice and specific to clinical context. The style of assessment associated with use of tools is one of direct assessment in using questions rather than more indirectly through observation and picking up patient/client cues that lead to illuminating conversation.

Research that considers aspects of spirituality in relation to health and social care contexts often uses a battery of tools rather than one that is singularly spiritually focused.[45] Inclusion of data that reflect psychological, social and physical functioning alongside tools to collect data concerning the spiritual dimension affirms the holistic nature of persons and that these aspects of humanity overlap (*see* Figure 1.1). In a review of literature that explored how research on the concept of spirituality had been reported across the decade 1990 to 2000, Chiu *et al.*[18] found that most qualitative studies used research instruments measuring the degree of one or more attributes of spirituality. The most frequently used instrument was one of established reliability and validity, which was Paloutzian and Ellison's[7] Spiritual Well-being Scale. This is a Likert-style scale consisting of 20 items that express spirituality in terms of religious wellbeing alternated with those of existential wellbeing (see examples above). A second popular instrument was The Spiritual Orientation Inventory (SOI).[46] Based on humanistic philosophy, it was designed to measure the spirituality of the non-religious and consists of 85 items that measure nine distinct spiritual attributes (Box 3.2).

Box 3.2 SOI nine spiritual attributes[46]

1 Transcendent dimension
2 Meaning and purpose
3 Mission in life
4 Sacredness of life
5 Material values
6 Altruism
7 Idealism
8 Awareness of the tragic
9 Fruits of spirituality

If 'spiritual assessment', rather than gathering information concerning a patient's spirituality,[37] is to be a practice focus to fulfil requirements of governance and audit, the tool to initiate/achieve this needs to be succinct if it is to be easy to use and not time-consuming to complete. Research instruments are inclined to range from lengthy, as in the first example above, to excessively long, exemplified in the second example, and therefore not suitable for use in practice environments. Similarly, research utilises tools that measure spirituality in relation to the focus of the study chosen, for example the non-religious in using the SOI instrument. Practice tools need to be balanced and reflect assessment of potential religious, sacred and secular spiritual need. Therefore, research instruments are generally of limited use in practice contexts.

Assessment tools in published literature vary in style and consider spiritual assessment in healthcare settings. There are a number that are of American origin. Stoll[47] was one of the earliest to publish suggested questions for assessment of spiritual need, but questions are religious in focus. Hungelmann et al.[48] produced the JAREL Spiritual Well-Being Scale in a style similar to Paloutzian and Ellison's scale,[7] constituting on this occasion 21 questions of both a religious and non-religious nature. Designed to facilitate care by diagnosing patient/client position on the spiritual continuum of 'potential for enhanced spiritual wellbeing' or 'spiritual distress' (p.265), it proved of limited or potentially limited use in a number of patient/client groups; the depressed, stressed, angry and confused found the Likert scale difficult to use and there were also problems with older adults with visual or hearing deficits, and potential issues for use in acute settings because of the physical or mental status of patients. Lengthy tools also demand concentration, which is often lacking during periods of illness. A third example of an American assessment tool is that of Dossey,[33] the purpose of which was to 'assist in assessing, evaluating, and increasing awareness of spirituality in yourselves and others' (p.46). This comprehensive set of questions has already been considered for its potential use in relation to personal spirituality (see above). However, it is very lengthy and would be time-consuming if used in a clinical context. It is a tool that includes both religious and non-religious perspectives of spirituality, but the nature and style of questions are potentially intrusive or intimidating when using with others within English culture(s).

A British publication by Govier[49] outlines 'five Rs of spirituality' as a foundation for assessment of spiritual needs. These are reason, reflection, religion, relationships and restoration (Table 3.3).

Table 3.3 The 'five Rs of spirituality'[49]

Reason and Reflection	The search for meaning in life experiences
Religion	As a vehicle for expressing spirituality
Relationships	With self, others and God
Restoration	Positive influence on physical dimension of person

He offers guidance for spiritual assessment by giving examples of observations or questions for each 'R' and using further questions to develop patient/client initial responses. Govier[49] implies that his assessment guidelines are unsuitable for patients in acute areas or day wards, where interaction is brief or limited, and better for continuing care or rehabilitation units where patients spend sufficient time to explore spiritual issues. However, McCord et al.'s[50] study suggests that spiritual inquiry should be directed towards individuals who suffer serious illness. Serious illness in acute settings can result in patients asking ultimate questions and questioning the meaning of their past life. Although stay may be relatively short, serious illness can result in an intensity of rapport between patient, their significant others and professionals that may result in these or similar guidelines being of value to professionals in developing use of appropriate questions to clarify the spiritual needs of patients. Similarly, regular patient and staff encounter in day wards may provide relationships in which clients/patients might feel confident to confide their most intimate spiritual concerns, for example in hospice day care.

Hodge[51] published a tool for spiritual assessment in social care contexts. He advocates the use of spiritual lifemaps as 'a client-centred pictorial instrument for spiritual assessment' (p.77). He acknowledges that clients can become so stuck in present, often chronic, difficulties that they overlook potential to resolve obstacles, and believes that assessment using lifemaps provides the means for exploring how individuals have dealt with past challenges and identifies strengths that exist in the person's spirituality.

Catterall et al.[52] audited the effectiveness of spiritual care provided for patients. In order to achieve this they devised a spiritual care standard that included initial assessment and ongoing review of the spiritual health and care needs of patients. McSherry and Ross[42] point out that development of such standards suggests spirituality is firmly on the healthcare agenda but encourage caution when evaluating data from audit. They refer to the lack of common understanding of the 'jargon surrounding spirituality' (p.484) as an example of a problem affecting the quality of data. This problem with terminology is exemplified by Taylor,[53] who found that including the term 'need' after the word 'spiritual' impeded responses in a study concerning the spiritual needs of patients with cancer.

Unpublished tools, developed in practice and specific to clinical context, also vary in style. Some are produced as a flow chart identifying whether the patient is religious or not, and then move on to the appropriate set of questions regarding needs. However, the questions delineated to each category may not be mutually exclusive. Alternatively, tools may combine spiritual assessment with psychosocial and cultural assessment. In these circumstances, it is easy for the professional to be distracted by assessing the most obvious need and circumventing the more difficult to discern. A more flexible option is the use of a set of guidelines outlining examples of questions that might be used, and consideration of how assessment might take place. Assessment tools are often used in the first instance when client/patients are admitted to a care context and would normally identify practical needs of spirituality, for example religious practice needs or the requirements of activities that are found to be uplifting, for example having access to a means of listening to music. Their inclusion in admission documentation affirms spirituality as a dimension of care that needs consideration. However, they are of little value unless the professional can interpret questions using terminology that the patient understands. Their success is dependent on how the assessment is performed and is reliant on the sensitivity and empathy of the professional using the tool.[35]

Spirituality is multidimensional and therefore it is not the prerogative of any one of the professions to assess the spiritual needs of patients. In reality, if assessment tools are to be used in this initial assessment, it is usually undertaken by a member of the professional group with the greatest contact with the patient/client. In institutional healthcare settings, for example, this would normally be a nurse. Whether assessment is direct in using a tool to question, or indirect in observation or within conversations as part of an established rapport, it is important for all carers to understand their personal and professional boundaries in relation to the spirituality of others. Therefore, another important facet in assessment of spiritual need is determining when it is appropriate to refer the need for further assessment to others.

Conclusion

Spiritual health is achievable even in circumstances of serious illness. Taking responsibility for spiritually healthy choices advocated by Booth[8] needs to be understood in relation to the limits of the human ability to control circumstances within the universal order. Spiritual maturity and the ability to be real is a lengthy process that may provide a resource that is as 'hidden as wisdom' (Merton, cited,[54] p.135) but may manifest itself as accommodative coping in ageing.

Spiritual intelligence is linked to personality and life circumstances and provides the means of achieving spiritual health. The need to seek and find meaning in suffering and hardship is spiritual, and a failure to do so may result in spiritual distress. In order to assess spiritual need in others, professionals need to be aware of their own spirituality.

For professionals experienced in the art of care, assessment of spiritual need emanates from observation, active listening and dialogue as part of an established and ongoing rapport with the client/patient. For the less experienced, tools can provide a source of guidance in spiritual assessment but should not be used as an instrument of interrogation. The inclusion of a spiritual assessment tool in admission documentation acknowledges spirituality as a dimension of care and initiates assessment of need. The value of assessment of client/patient spiritual need is in the identification of care that will be beneficial in contributing to their spiritual health.

References

1　Greenstreet W (1999) Teaching spirituality in nursing: a literature review. *Nurse Education Today*. **19**: 649–58.
2　Whitehead D (2003) Beyond the metaphysical: health-promoting existential mechanisms and their impact on the health status of clients. *Journal of Clinical Nursing*. **12**(5): 678–88.
3　Mohan K (2004) Eastern perspectives and implications for the West. In: Jewell A (ed.) *Ageing, Spirituality and Well-Being*. Jessica Kingsley, London.
4　Diener E, Suh E, Lucas R *et al.* (1999) Well-being: three decades of progress. *Psychological Bulletin*. **125**(2): 276–302.
5　Roy K (1979) Elements of mysticism in spiritual health. In: Moberg DO (ed.) *Spiritual Well-being: sociological perspectives*. University Press of America, Washington, DC.
6　Fehring RJ, Miller JF, Shaw C (1997) Spiritual well-being, religiosity, hope, depression, and other mood states in elderly people coping with cancer. *ONF*. **4**(4): 663–71.
7　Paloutzian RF, Ellison CW (1982) Loneliness: spiritual well being, and the quality of life. In: Peplau LA, Perlman D (eds) *Loneliness: a sourcebook of current theory, research and therapy*. John Wiley, New York, NY.
8　Booth L (1995) A new understanding of spirituality. *Journal of Chemical Dependency*. **5**(2): 5–17.
9　Williams M (1985) *The Velveteen Rabbit*. Avon Books, New York.
10　Pierce DE (2003) *Occupation by Design; Building Therapeutic Power*. FA Davies, Philadelphia, PA.
11　Zohar D, Marshall I (2000) *Spiritual Intelligence, the Ultimate Intelligence*. Bloomsbury, London.
12　Friedemann M, Mouch J, Racey T (2002) Nursing the spirit: the framework of systemic organization. *Journal of Advanced Nursing*. **39**(4): 325–32.
13　Espeland K (1999) Achieving spiritual wellness using reflective questions. *Journal of Psychosocial Nursing*. **37**(7): 36–40.
14　Diener E, Fujita F (1995) Resources, personal strivings, and subjective well-being: a nomothetic and idiographic approach. *Journal of Personality and Social Psychology*. **68**: 926–35.
15　Landis BJ (1996) Uncertainty, spiritual well-being and psychosocial adjustment to chronic illness. *Issues in Mental Health Nursing*. **17**: 217–31.
16　Daaleman TP, Kuckelman Cobb A, Frey BB (2001) Spirituality and well-being: an exploratory study of patient perspective. *Social Science and Medicine*. **53**: 1503–11.
17　Royal College of Nursing (2000) Spiritual intelligence. *Leader. The RCN Newsletter for Nurses Working in Management*. **Spring**: 6.
18　Chiu L, Emblen J, Van Hofwegen L *et al.* (2004) An integrated review of the concept of spirituality in the health sciences. *Western Journal of Nursing Research*. **26**(4): 405–28.
19　Fowler JW (1981) *Stages of Faith: the psychology of human development and the quest for meaning*. Harper and Row, Philadelphia, PA.
20　Kellehear A (2000) Spirituality and palliative care: a model of needs. *Palliative Medicine*. **14**(2): 149–55.
21　Murray SA, Kendall M, Boyd K *et al.* (2004) Exploring the spiritual needs of people dying of lung cancer or heart failure: a prospective qualitative interview study of patients and their carers. *Palliative Medicine*. **18**: 39–45.
22　Sheldrake P (1987) *Images of Holiness: explorations in contemporary spirituality*. Darton, Longman and Todd, London.
23　Whipp M (1998) Spirituality and the scientific mind: a dilemma for doctors. In: Cobb M, Robshaw V (eds) *The Spiritual Challenge of Health Care*. Churchill Livingstone, Edinburgh.
24　O'Brien ME (1982) The need for spiritual integrity. In: Yura H, Walsh MB (eds) *Human Needs and Nursing Process*. Appleton-Century-Crofts, Norwalk, Connecticut.
25　Jarvis P (1993) Meaning being and learning. In: Jarvis P, Walters N (eds) *Adult Education and Theological Interpretations*. Krieger, Malabar, Florida.
26　Twycross R (1999) *Introducing Palliative Care*. Radcliffe Medical Press, Oxford.
27　Watson J (1988) *Nursing: human science and human care, a theory of nursing*. National League of Nursing, New York, NY.

28 Hood Morris EL (1996) A spiritual well-being model: use with older women who experience depression. *Issues in Mental Health Nursing*. **17**: 439–55.

29 O'Reilly ML (2004) Spirituality and mental health clients. *Journal of Psychosocial Nursing and Mental Health Services*. **42**(7): 44–53.

30 Cornette K (1997) For whenever I am weak I am strong... *International Journal of Palliative Nursing*. **3**(1): 6–13.

31 Narayanasamy A, Gates B, Swinton J (2002) Spirituality and learning disabilities: a qualitative study. *British Journal of Nursing*. **11**(14): 948–57.

32 Pesut B (2003) Developing spirituality in the curriculum: worldviews, intrapersonal connectedness, interpersonal connectedness. *Nursing Education Perspective*. **24**(6): 290–4.

33 Dossey B (1998) Spiritual assessment tool. *American Journal of Nursing*. **98**(6): 46.

34 Hermann M (2003) Keeping the magic alive in nursing care: advice from the Dalai Lama. *Nurse Educator*. **28**(6): 245–6.

35 Swinton J, Narayanasamy A (2002) Response to 'A critical view of spirituality and spiritual assessment'. *Journal of Advanced Nursing*. **40**(2): 158–60.

36 Speck P, Higginson I, Addington-Hall J (2004) Spiritual needs in health care. *BMJ*. **329**: 123–4.

37 Pierpont JH (2003) Spiritual assessment. *Social Work*. **48**(4): 562–3.

38 Narayanasamy A, Clisset P, Parumal L *et al.* (2004) Responses to the spiritual needs of older people. *Journal of Advanced Nursing*. **48**(1): 6–16.

39 Froggatt K (1997) Signposts on the journey: the place of ritual in spiritual care. *International Journal of Palliative Nursing*. **3**(1): 42–6.

40 Carson VB (1989) Spirituality and the nursing process. In: Carson VB (ed.) *Spiritual Dimensions of Nursing Practice*. Saunders, Philadelphia, PA.

41 Draper P, McSherry W (2002) A critical view of spirituality and spiritual assessment. *Journal of Advanced Nursing*. **39**(1): 1–2.

42 McSherry W, Ross L (2002) Dilemmas of spiritual assessment: considerations for nursing practice. *Journal of Advanced Nursing*. **38**(5): 479–88.

43 Walter T (1994) *The Revival of Death*. Routledge, London.

44 Bash A (2004) Spirituality; the emperor's new clothes? *Journal of Clinical Nursing*. **13**(1): 11–16.

45 McClain CS, Rosenfeld B, Breitbart W (2003) Effect of spiritual well-being on end-of-life despair in terminally-ill cancer patients. *The Lancet*. **361**: 1603–7.

46 Elkins DN, Hedstrom LJ, Hughes LL *et al.* (1988) Toward a humanistic-phenomenological spirituality. *Journal of Humanistic Psychology*. **28**(4): 5–18.

47 Stoll R (1979) Guidelines for a spiritual assessment. *American Journal of Nursing*. **79**: 1574–7.

48 Hungelmann J, Kenkel-Rossi E, Klassen L *et al.* (1996) Focus on spiritual well-being: harmonious interconnectedness of mind-body-spirit- use of the JAREL Spiritual Well-Being Scale. *Geriatric Nursing*. **17**(6): 262–6.

49 Govier I (2000) Spiritual care in nursing: a systematic approach. *Nursing Standard*. **14**(17): 32–6.

50 McCord G, Gilchrist VJ, Grossman SD *et al.* (2004) Discussing spirituality with patients: a rational and ethical approach. *Annals of Family Medicine*. **2**: 356–61.

51 Hodge DR (2005) Spiritual lifemaps: a client-centred pictorial instrument for spiritual assessment, planning, and intervention. *Social Work*. **50**(1): 77–87.

52 Catterall RA, Cox M, Greet B *et al.* (1998) The assessment and audit of spiritual care. *International Journal of Palliative Nursing*. **4**: 162–8.

53 Taylor EJ (2003) Spiritual needs of patients with cancer and family caregivers. *Cancer Nursing*. **26**(4): 260–6.

54 Dumont C (1974) The contemplative. In: Hart P (ed.) *Thomas Merton, Monk, A Monastic Tribute*. Hodder and Stoughton, London.

Spiritual care in health and social care settings

CHAPTER 4

Spiritual care

Wendy Greenstreet

Introduction

Holistic philosophy affirms spirituality as a valid component of care. However, it is important not to view spirituality as the 'emperor's new clothes'[1] (p.15), attributing the concept an objective reality that does not exist. It is a myriad of subjective possibilities, each person consciously or unconsciously formulating their own spiritual co-ordinates as an expression of their humanity.[1] Consequently, spiritual care needs to reflect a kaleidoscope of options from which a pattern of care that mirrors patient need emanates. If clients/patients have their own means of fulfilling their spiritual needs then professional carers need not intrude further unless circumstances change. The spiritual dimension of a person transcends and holds together the biopsychosocial (*see* Figures 1.1 and 1.2). Therefore, spiritual care is integral to and not separate from other aspects of care. Assessment of need on admission to health and social care contexts may well identify practical aspects of care that need to be arranged or provided. This generates activity that constitutes 'doing' in relation to spiritual care.

However, much of spiritual care relies, as does ongoing assessment of need, on the relationship between professional and client/patient, on the nature of the carer's ability to 'be with' the individual in the delivery of care. Collectively, spiritual care is about healing rather than cure, 'wholeness' rather than recovery. The chapter ends in considering issues in spiritual care; who should be involved in spiritual care is a potential source of controversy, although there appears to be some consensus on the barriers that limit its provision.

'Doing' and spiritual care

Generally the activity of 'doing' by health and social care professionals involved in spiritual care either constitutes facilitating client/patient practices that they find spiritually uplifting or referral to others who have specialist skills that can help those in spiritual need.

Religious practice and rituals

For those who have a religious faith, the practice of religious ritual can be a source of consolation during ill health or difficult circumstances. Professionals need to facilitate access to the means of fulfilling this need and respect client/patient religious and cultural preference when planning care. In a multicultural society, health and social care professionals need to have a general awareness of the practices of different world religions to enable them to do this. Summaries of cultural and religious practice for professional carers are available in published sources, for example Neuberger,[2] Green,[3,4] Narayanasamy,[5] but are also produced by professional practitioners for use in specific healthcare trusts, institutions or practice contexts. Gunaratnam[6] refers to these as factfiles and acknowledges their value in meeting professional needs for guidance and information in relation to task-oriented practice issues. However, she warns that, in classifying beliefs and practices in sweeping generalisations, these factfiles may result in crude stereotyping of religious practice. It is important for professional carers not to interpret these prescriptively but engage in dialogue with those in their care regarding their idiosyncratic interpretation of religion and the consequent implications for care.

Facilitation of rites, sacraments and client/patient need to discuss religious concerns may require the involvement of their religious community and/or its leader. Alternatively, most healthcare institutions employ a chaplain, whose remit is one of pastoral care rather than a focused denominational role, who could support those having different religious faiths and offer spiritual guidance. This broader remit may also mean that a chaplain can provide a source of support for the non-religious in discussing wider spiritual issues that are causing concern rather than those of a religious nature. However, the public image of a chaplain is one associated with religion, therefore patients/clients with no faith may decline this opportunity of referral.

Prayer is primarily associated with religious practice, but even those who do not profess a religious faith have been known to pray in some situations.[7] Prayer as a means of conversing with God provides clients/patients with a source of coping in times of duress.[8] The challenge in institutional settings is to achieve an ambience to allow prayer; peace and privacy, which can be elusive in the bustle of clinical environments. Carers who do not share a client/patient's faith can feel uncomfortable when asked to participate in prayer or read religious literature. However, it is important to differentiate between reading and belief. Staying with a client/patient while they pray, or reading to them, does not imply belief but evidence of a supportive relationship. An understanding of personal spirituality will help professionals acknowledge the different beliefs of others without demeaning or imposing their own.

Dietary and other cultural requirements associated with religious practice are discussed in Chapter 9.

Creative therapy, music, art and spiritual counselling

As spirituality, in its interpretation as a wider phenomenon than religion, has gained credibility as a significant perspective of health and social care, the role of the more creative forms of therapy has also been acknowledged in meeting the needs of spiritual care where empirical knowledge has fallen short. William James, exploring the varieties of religious experience at the beginning of the twentieth century, was already identifying the value of 'healthy-mindedness as a religious attitude'[9] (p.90) and giving examples of those without religious faith valuing 'lively songs and music ... nature, especially fine weather' (p.93) as evidence of the gathering momentum of what he called the 'Mind-cure movement' (p.94).

Kaptchuk[10] writes of the contemporary appeal of alternative medicine in its advocacy of spirituality, offering 'empowerment, authenticity, and enlarged self-identity when illness threatens their sense of intactness and connection to the world' (p.1061). Spirituality in this context is associated with healing care rather than with curative treatment. The term 'healing' is derived from Saxon and German words for 'whole' in being more than freedom from difficulty or symptoms and more to do with care attending to meaning, value and purpose that underpin human experience.[11] Similarly, Wright[12] describes healing 'as concerned not so much with a change in a particular illness but rather with a change in consciousness – our way of being with it... Healing has a deeper resonance concerning an emotional and spiritual transformation in which bodily changes and the resolution of disease may or may not happen' (p.14). It is a potential within all of us at all times.[13] This contemporary return to an interest in healing is perhaps symbolic of a new discourse that does not polarise the art and science of care but holds both in balance, with the equilibrium determined by the circumstances of situation.

Conventional forms of scientific measurement are unable to identify the benefits of spiritual therapies. Therefore, those who look for a scientific evidence base for all care view such therapies with scepticism. However, the traditional forms of spiritual therapy have endured the test of time. Traditional therapies stem from religious and humanistic views. They tend to target spiritual problems resulting from a situation,[14] for example pain due to the loss of a loved one. Therapies include music, prayer, contemplation, receiving religious rites and spiritual counselling.

The 'New Age' approach to spiritual therapy differs. The intention is to use therapy of a spiritual nature to focus on dealing with the disorder or disease itself.[14] An example might be in the use of therapeutic touch which centres on altering a patient's energy field. The disorder or disease would be seen as a depletion within an individual's energy field, so therapy would aim to correct the imbalance in energy and resolve the disorder or disease. Other examples of New Age therapies include relaxation, guided imagery and aromatherapy.

Some traditional and New Age therapies appear similar. An example is the New Age therapy of therapeutic touch and the traditional equivalent of the laying on of hands. Barnum[14] explains that it is not the techniques that differ but the motivation of these therapies. The laying on of hands is seen as conveying God's power through the healer. Therapeutic touch channels universal power through the therapist to the patient. Universal power is described as the forces of nature,[15] rather than a personalised God.

Music allows both spiritual and emotional release.[8] It can be interpreted in the light of past experiences and may well have proved spiritually uplifting at other similarly difficult times.[16] Different types of music have different effects on mood[17] and can, for example, reduce anxiety, alleviate depression and energise the spirit.[8] Music as a means of promoting wellbeing is discussed further in Chapter 12.

Purposeful activity such as creative art, structured work and enjoying nature are further elements of spiritual care[11] and are explored further in Chapters 10 and 11. Creative arts can assist humanity to see itself by mirroring the human experience.

They provide 'authentic, human forms of uncovering experience and open up the subjective in ways that generate insight and understanding'[18] (p.46).

The spiritually distressed might benefit from specialist counselling. Basic counselling skills are normally included in professional pre-registration inter-personal skills tuition.[19] However, counselling those who are unable to invest life with meaning requires specialist skills. Brody *et al.*[20] believe that spiritual counsellors should be able to understand and be conversant with the biomedical aspects of a case but not necessarily be physicians, have had training in psychology but not necessarily be psychologists, and should be skilled in the understanding of human relationships and able to 'integrate the personal meanings of values for both themselves and their patients' (p.204). Burnard[21] suggests a slightly different but equally exacting list of experience necessary for counselling the spiritually distressed. These include:

- wide reading to ensure an appreciation of how 'ultimate' questions of life have been approached by past religious, philosophical and political thinkers
- a highly developed intuitive sense enabling understanding beyond the words clients/patients use to express themselves
- clarity of beliefs
- thorough skills training in listening and questioning techniques backed by considerable life experience
- an understanding and use of approaches to help patients with emotional release
- an awareness that there are no ready answers to many of the questions that are likely to be raised.

Should the less experienced try to counsel the spiritually distressed, they may well compound their patients' problems or even lose their own way and need help themselves.

Creative therapy and spiritual counselling for clients/patients involves referral to skilled practitioners. Although some health and social care professionals may have the skills to teach patients simple relaxation, for example, or facilitate access to music, their primary role is to be aware of the sources of creative therapy and counselling available to their client/patient group and refer individuals with identified spiritual needs appropriately.

'Being' and spiritual care

Spiritual care is not just about facilitation of activity but engaging with those in receipt of health or social care who are trying to make sense of the circumstances they find themselves in, in their search for answers to ultimate questions.[11,22,23] This engagement requires a sharing of the self in a way of 'being' that reflects the art of care. The professional carer's attitude to and the nature of the relationships with clients/patients requires a number of personal qualities that include sensitivity in communication, 'moderated love', confidence, an ability to engender hope and 'hearing' expression of the spiritual in metaphor and narrative.

Being present

Sensitivity of communication is conveyed in compassionate authenticity[24] and moves physical 'presence' of professional carers 'being there' for clients/patients onto 'being with' the patient psychologically.[25] Spiritual matters are by nature intimate and so they are more likely to be raised within a relationship of genuineness and trust. Such discussion can never be organised or planned but happens spontaneously when the ambience is right for the patient. Individuals often do not reveal their personal thoughts in a direct manner, but allude to them in a roundabout way, not revealing too much of themselves too soon.[26] In order to 'hear' what is being said, professional carers need to actively listen, giving their whole attention to picking up and pursuing clues the client/patient gives, including body language. Clients/patients need the opportunity to express their uncertainties, not necessarily expecting answers, and those providing a supportive 'presence' need to accept and be honest with those in their care by owning that for some questions there are no answers. O'Reilly[27] refers to professional's use of self in 'being with' others as a therapeutic means of alleviation of suffering, personal growth through difficult experiences and a reduced sense of isolation.

Breaking through the barriers of objectivity

Spiritual care needs to be offered without preconditions; each individual must be valued, accepted where they are with their own needs and attitudes. Stoter[28] refers to such care as a gift of love. Campbell[29] believes that members of personal service professions provide 'consistent, skilled and informed concern' (p.6). He describes the balance needed to achieve informed concern as 'moderated love', which falls between an absence or an excess of professional detachment. Both Morse et al.[30] and Campbell[29] contribute to discussion on how nurses can reveal the essence of what is meant by a balanced professional relationship in relation to spiritual care. However, the principles conveyed within these discussions are applicable to other health and social care professions. For example, Van Amburg[31] believes that occupational therapy is hindered by the ethical consideration of maintaining objective client-therapist relationships. Objectivity is seen as a disengaged perspective that depersonalises human relationships when meaningful experiences 'require engaged, sympathetic relationships to be spiritually manifested' (p.186). Similarly, Cassell[32] encourages physicians to take a less objective stance in allowing patients to experience something of who they are as helpful in diagnosing suffering and identifying patients fears, interpretation of meaning and concerns for the future regarding symptoms.

Morse et al.[30] describe four types of communication patterns that reflect expressions of caring. Group categories are determined by communication that is either patient-focused or self-focused and responses that are either reflexive or learned (Figure 4.1).

Professionals who focus on self, either reflexively or as a learned response, and are therefore disengaged or detached to protect themselves from suffering, are unable to contribute to spiritual care. Learned responses that are patient-focused but limit personal investment in suffering that demands emotional labour[33] are relatively detached, objective and described as professional in nature. Therapeutically

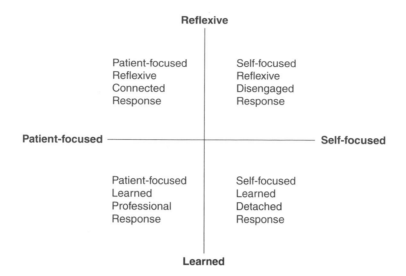

Figure 4.1 Communication patterns reflecting expressions of caring.[30]

'at arm's length'[30] (p.816) professionals dutifully 'care for' clients/patients by trying to imagine a patient's experience rather than becoming genuinely involved. This style of communication does not facilitate spiritual care either.

Communication that expresses spiritual caring is sourced from a style that to some extent predates professional learning and is one that professionals may need to open themselves to once again. Reflexive responses are patient-focused and triggered by the emotional insight of the carer. Culturally conditioned rather than learned, these responses provide a natural source of comfort to clients/patients. It is perhaps this human response to another's suffering that accounts for the support clients/patients find in conversations with non-professionals in health and social care settings. A critical factor in this level of response is that the care giver is emotionally involved or 'connected' and able to identify with the sufferer. Immersion in another's reality results in sharing the experience of suffering. This 'caring about' another demands energy and strength that is the emotional labour described by James.[33]

Campbell[29] also implies that emotional involvement is necessary for caring and suggests companionship as the means of achieving 'moderated' love. Such a balanced professional relationship with clients/patients provides a vehicle to effect spiritual care. A 'good companion' (p.49) shares the route, does not impose, but allows clients/patients to make their chosen journey. Components of companionship of this kind include closeness without sexual stereotyping, movement onward, mutuality and commitment within defined limits.

Closeness extends the description of 'presence' as one that is not gender related. Sensing and accommodating patient need would be central to such closeness. This might be exemplified by physical care given with patience and attentiveness, conveying care as loving without any need for exchange of words. In helping patients move onwards, whether towards recovery or death, the professional companion can use their experience to encourage clients/patients in moments when they feel lost. Mutuality within companionship affirms 'being with' the patient. Campbell[29] points out the high cost to human resources of a constant presence with illness and the sharing of suffering. The commitment of companionship is limited in that it arises incidentally due to the client/patient's circumstances and ends at the journey's destination, either recovery or death. Campbell[29] believes this to be beneficial to both professional carer and patient, who each have their own lives to lead. He sees the professional whose life outside the caring environment has its own richness as being more able to achieve a balanced relationship with patients, and therefore finding it easier to 'let go' at the journey's end. Parting can be painful, but support from others who have shared caring for the patient can help resolve the sense of loss. Also, reflection on the journey shared with the patient can help the professional acknowledge any personal growth that has resulted from companionship that they have to offer future patients.

Confidence

The implication of personal involvement in spiritual care requires confidence. Clarity regarding personal spiritual awareness helps engender the confidence needed to enable professionals to stay with the vulnerable asking unanswerable questions. Knowledge of the art that is spiritual care is both tacit and intuitive, and so learnt experientially rather than taught. Confidence grows as professionals come to trust intuitive thinking that comes out of reflective processing of experience until ultimately they are able to feel client/patient feelings.[32] Life experiences also contribute to this confidence.[34] Personal crises can act as a force for growth towards self-actualisation, a quality that tolerates uncertainty and appreciates others unconditionally. Hence, such growth is not necessarily associated with chronological age or length of time in professional practice.

The role of hope

Hope as an aspect of spirituality enables creativity. In conveying a sense of future, hope contributes to the purpose of life ahead. During illness, hope may be sustained by trusting in the 'cure' available. However, for those who suffer from a disease for which there is no cure, a change in perspective is needed from one of 'dying from a terminal illness to living with a life threatening illness'[35] (p.661). Therefore hope is a potential motivator moving people towards new options and alternative ways of coping. Hope, rather than a sense of future in relation to cure, becomes a sense of future in relation to quality of life left.[36] Exploration of the concept of hope and strategies to engender hope are discussed in Chapter 5.

Recognising the expression of the spiritual

The client/patient intuitively uses metaphor, symbol and narrative to express experiences for which there is no common intellectual language. Metaphorical language is symbolic. It attempts to explain the unfamiliar by referring to the familiar without suggesting the two are literally the same.[37] The subjective experience of spirituality is diluted or lost in conventional rational expression. However, metaphor creates an image that illuminates the expression of matters of spirituality both for those who recount them and those who listen. Stanworth[38] argues that symbol and metaphor are the tools of story making.

Narrative and the search for meaning

> To narrate experience is to retell it in a certain way for a certain end.[39]
> (p.556)

Narrative provides a means of refashioning biography in the search to make sense of current circumstances as serious illness, or difficulties, undermine personhood and an individual's roles in the world.[38] Narrative unifies past experiences, so the past is not thought of as lost but as something we can never leave behind. Recounting stories of the past helps articulation and understanding of present problems and so impacts action directed towards the future.[39] Larner[39] refers to narratives as reflecting life as lived forwards while understood backwards, and to how 'stories of the past act as containers for the seeds of change in the future' (p.550). Pearson et al.[18] compares different approaches to narrative that are concerned with different topics and demonstrates that, in all cases, the meaning that comes out of illness is as significant as the objective disease state itself or its social consequences.

Becker[40] explains that not all client/patient narratives are coherent. Chronic illness can produce chaotic stories that miss a beginning and an end; illness continuously destroys or threatens the self so every narrative of the ill self remains fragile. Becker[40] illustrates the art of listening to and interpreting narrative. She compares patient narratives that did not follow a chronological pattern.

The first narrative was confusing and contradictory. She owns that she initially doubted the patient's narrative competence. As Becker became accustomed to the way the person told her story she recognised a poetic quality to the patient's account and how the 'circularity and the repetition of certain phrases increased the effect' (p.77). Here the narrative was poetic, and coherence and meaning flowed from its organisation in verses.[41] This repetition and poetic style of narrative is referred to by other authors;[18,39] the 're-peats' being of potentialities inherited from the past[39] (p.556).

A second example was a patient whose initial narrative was scientific, ordered, having a beginning, middle and end. However, after relating his tale, the patient did not know whether the events he recounted had caused his pain. In asking how he felt about his pain, Becker found that he recounted a very different style of story that was not integrated and coherent. He had, therefore, demonstrated different ways of talking that seemed to be unconnected. He could not tell a conventional chronological story that implied both the cause of his pain and his feelings.

Becker's account illustrates the need for professional carers to persevere in listening to narrative that is repetitive and repeated and not to expect ordered stories. Allowing narrative, acknowledging its value by attending to what is said, is important. Patients are not necessarily describing or re-describing experiences or their deepest beliefs, but may actually be searching for or refining their understanding as they recount their story.[38]

Issues in spiritual care

Who should be involved in spiritual care?

King[42] explains that health and social science disciplines are all concerned with the same stream of life experience but reduce it differently because each has a different focus of attention that comes from their different purposes. She advocates that transdisciplinary approaches are beneficial and reflect controversies between disciplines as mainly issues of emphasis. However, a shift in emphasis within the same discipline can have a significant impact on actual care delivered.

Traditionally, the primary focus of care for chaplains employed within health and social care has been religious support. However, increasingly, they have a pastoral role, with a wider remit of care related to spirituality. In representing a medical perspective, Culliford[43] refers to the increasing recognition of the importance of spiritual values and skills in clinical care and suggests spiritual sustenance is as crucial to healing as nutrition. However, Kliewer[44] refers to resistance by physicians who challenge the premise of integrating spiritual and medical care, claiming that it 'trivializes a deep and complex reality'. McColl[45] exemplifies the view of many who support spirituality as an aspect of occupational therapy, but Mayers[46] accepts that therapists may feel uncomfortable in discussing spiritual issues with clients, and Whalley Hammell[47] proposes abandoning the term 'spirituality' in occupational therapy altogether. Most nursing literature reflects spiritual care as a nursing responsibility.[48,49] However, Draper and McSherry[50] propose that a significant proportion of people do not know what the term spirituality means or do not believe that their lives have a spiritual dimension so that universalising the concept as an aspect of nursing care may attribute a value to clients/patients that they do not share. The dearth of literature conveying any view of spirituality within radiography reflects the technical focus of its code of professional practice, but comment by those writing from a social work perspective acknowledge spirituality as an important, albeit as yet relatively unexplored, area within their discipline.[51]

Regardless of professional debate, it is not a matter of who ought to give spiritual care but a matter of who can.[52] Communication is at the heart of spiritual care. If clients/patients have a spiritual need (although they are unlikely to use this term), they will 'open up' to others they can trust. Established, warm relationships in which professionals of any discipline are able to be responsive in a way that Morse et al.[30] describe as fundamentally one of reflexive humanity, provide the conduit for clients/patients sharing concerns about their very being. As every client/patient is different and health and social care (ideally) involves interprofessional, multidisciplinary working,[52] who gets to 'hear', or is intuitively astute enough to recognise, an individual's spiritual need(s) will not be profession specific. However, professional purpose results in different patterns and duration of contact that may impact styles of rapport with client/patient groups and account for different levels of interest in the spiritual dimension of care, for example, between nursing and radiography. Regardless of profession, those who rely solely on professional, disengaged or detached styles of communication[30] are unlikely to be chosen by patients for intimation of need. Also, those professionals whose world-view does not acknowledge a spiritual dimension, who are not comfortable with or who lack confidence in understanding what is meant by this dimension of a person are unlikely to be able to provide spiritual care. The expression of need may in itself constitute the fulfilment of that need, the care in these instances comprising presence and attentive listening. However, spirituality is multifaceted and clients/patients may benefit from referral to other disciplines or professions. The insight and knowledge required to determine when this is necessary and decide appropriate referral also constitutes spiritual care.

Ethics and spiritual care

The vulnerability of clients/patients in health and social care settings makes the professional carer potentially more powerful within relationships in practice settings. It is therefore ethically imperative that professionals are clear that it is the patient's spiritual beliefs that drive this dimension of care and not their own.[44]

Collaboration with the client/patient balances power and promotes ethical practice. Daaleman[53] exemplifies how this can be achieved in medicine. He conceives spirituality to be the means by which a patient begins to integrate their illness experience within their life course and how well this meaning making empowers them to live their lives. As a physician, he owns that he implies the path of an illness by the clinical impression he conveys and the selection of therapeutic interventions offered, and so creates a cultural script of disease trajectory. To include spirituality as a perspective of care, he believes that this needs to shift to co-creation of a clinical narrative that includes the context of the patient's life course. He uses the example of a patient with cancer who felt depressed. In discussion, he came to understand that the patient saw the cancer as a threat to her ability to work and remain productive, a source of empowerment in her life, rather than it representing a death threat. Instead of just prescribing interventions for the disease, insight into the patient's understanding meant Daaleman[53] could work with his patient to define the nature of the best outcome that would allow her to live her life at that time. The principle of sharing professional expertise in an empowering relationship that allows clients/patients to express the meaning of their situation within their life context is ethical and facilitates spiritual care in a way that is relevant across health and social care professions. Newman[54] reflects a similar view in describing experiencing the 'whole' in nursing as:

> ...moving from attention on the other as object to attention to the we in relationship, from fixing things to attending to the meaning of the whole, from hierarchical one-way intervention to mutual process partnering. (p.36)

Confidentiality and documentation of information regarding spiritual care is an ethical issue.[55] Clients/patients should be involved in decisions about sharing information about their spiritual life or made aware of the necessity to do so. Both McSherry and Ross[55] and Farvis[56] acknowledge the need for some documentation to ensure communication between professional carers and continuity of care for clients/patients. However, as spiritual care largely takes the form of human interaction that is itself therapeutic,[56] if documentation is necessary it is limited to acknowledging the occurrence of such interaction but cannot reflect the personal language used in spiritual care.[57]

Barriers to spiritual care provision

One of the most fundamental barriers to spiritual care provision is personal to professional carers. The concern is either a failure to be in touch with personal spirituality or one of potentially projecting personal beliefs onto those in their care.[25,58,59] Some believe that spirituality is situation based and should only be addressed if the client/patient brings it up.[58] McCord *et al.*,[60] for example, found that age appeared to affect patient enthusiasm in spiritual discussion with their physicians. Others have identified a lack of time, experience and education,[55,58] or a lack of staff,[55] as issues that challenge the delivery of spiritual care.

Education, both in workshop activities[52,61] and educational programmes,[19,59,62] provide a safe context in which to explore and gain confidence in the provision of spiritual care. Encouragement to consider personal stance in relation to spirituality needs to be accompanied by examples of ways this may be achieved and why it is an important activity. Shared experiences can illustrate how care that falls outside personal belief might be approached. Discussion using anecdotes taken from practice can provide examples of who initiates spiritually focused conversation, and how 'additional' aspects of care can be attempted within time constraints and with staff shortages. If groups are multiprofessional, profession-specific issues can be explored interprofessionally. These groups also provide an opportunity to express and explore concerns of boundary violation.

Conclusion

Professional carers may have a key role in facilitating religious practice or access to available creative forms of therapy. This type of activity is easily described, and so possible to record. Similarly, whether such care is effected can be measured, although its effectiveness is more likely to be qualitatively rather than quantitatively expressed. The aspect of spiritual care that is more difficult to describe is more intuitive in nature. Sourced from experience and having the confidence to engage with the patient's vulnerability, the professional carer shares the experience of suffering in emotional labour. Such a relationship needs to remain balanced, as one of companionship. This entails commitment that arises incidentally from client/patient circumstances that have brought them into health or social care and ends in the resolution of hardship, recovery or death. Attending to narrative allows the client/patient to refashion their biography and refine their understanding of the meaning of their illness or difficulties. Who should provide spiritual care is a matter of who can, rather than being profession specific. Most professional carers could facilitate referral to allow the fulfilment of ritual or therapy, but not all understand the concept of spirituality in health and social care. Others might use only objective, disengaged or detached styles of communication that do not enable the provision of spiritual care. Education provides a means of overcoming barriers to spiritual care provision by raising personal and professional awareness of spirituality as a concept, and promoting an understanding of spirituality as a perspective of care.

References

1 Bash A (2004) Spirituality; the emperor's new clothes? *Journal of Clinical Nursing*. **13**(1): 11–16.

2 Neuberger J (1987) *Caring for Dying People of Different Faiths*. Austen Cornish, Lisa Sainsbury, London.

3 Green J (1991) *Death with Dignity: meeting the spiritual needs of patients in a multicultural society*. NT, London.

4 Green J (1993) *Death with Dignity: meeting the spiritual needs of patients in a multicultural society*, volume 2. NT, London.

5 Narayanasamy A (2001) *Spiritual Care: a practical guide for nurses and healthcare practitioners*. Quay, Dinton, Wiltshire.

6 Gunaratnam Y (1997) Culture is not enough: a critique of multi-culturalism in palliative care. In: Field D, Hockey J, Small N (eds) *Death, Gender and Ethnicity*. Routledge, London.

7 Sheldrake P (1987) *Images of Holiness: explorations in contemporary spirituality*. Darton, Longman and Todd, London.

8 Stoll RI (1989) Spirituality and chronic illness. In: Carson VB (ed.) *Spiritual Dimensions of Nursing Practice*. Saunders, Philadelphia, PA.

9 James W (1982) *The Varieties of Religious Experience*. Penguin, Harmondsworth, Middlesex.

10 Kaptchuk TJ (1998) The persuasive appeal of alternative medicine. *Annals of Internal Medicine*. **129**(12): 1061–5.

11 Culliford L (2002) Spiritual care and psychiatric treatment: an introduction. *Advances in Psychiatric Treatment*. **8**: 249–61.

12 Wright S (2005) Encouraging nature to act. *Nursing Standard*. **19**(17): 14–15.

13 Crombez J, Dubreucq J (1991) Can one die healed? *Journal of Palliative Care*. **7**(2): 39–43.

14 Barnum BS (1996) *Spirituality in Nursing, from Traditional to New Age*. Springer, New York, NY.

15 Bradshaw A (1994) *Lighting the Lamp, The Spiritual Dimension of Nursing Care*. Scutari Press, Harrow, Middlesex.

16 Ferszt G, Taylor PB (1988) When your patient needs spiritual comfort. *Nursing*. **18**(4): 48–9.

17 McCraty R, Barrios-Choplin B, Atkinson M *et al.* (1998) The effects of different types of music on mood, tension, and mental clarity. *Alternative Therapies*. **4**(1): 75–84.

18 Pearson A, Borbasi S, Walsh K (1997) Practicing nursing therapeutically through acting as a skilled companion on the illness journey. *Advanced Practice Nursing Quarterly*. **3**: 46–52.

19 Greenstreet W (1999) Teaching spirituality in nursing: a literature review. *Nurse Education Today*. **19**: 649–58.

20 Brody H, Jeffery L, Cardinal MA *et al.* (2004) Addressing spiritual concerns in family medicine: a team approach. *The Journal of the American Board of Family Practice*. **17**: 201–6.

21 Burnard P (1987) Spiritual distress and the nursing response: theoretical considerations and counselling skills. *Journal of Advanced Nursing*. **12**: 377–82.

22 Lunt A (2001) The roots of recovery. *Journal of Psychosocial Nursing and Mental Health Services*. **39**(11): 48–50.

23 Speck P, Higginson I, Addington-Hall J (2004) Spiritual needs in healthcare. *BMJ*. **329**: 123–4.

24 Golberg B (1998) Connection: an exploration of spirituality in nursing care. *Journal of Advanced Nursing*. **27**(4): 836–42.

25 Davidhizar R (2000) The spiritual needs of hospitalised patients. *American Journal of Nursing*. **100**(7): 24C–24D.

26 Carson VB (1989) Spirituality and the nursing process. In: Carson VB (ed.) *Spiritual Dimensions of Nursing Practice*. Saunders, Philadelphia, PA.

27 O'Reilly ML (2004) Spirituality and mental health clients. *Journal of Psychosocial Nursing and Mental Health Services*. **42**(7): 44–53.

28 Stoter D (1995) *Spiritual Aspects of Health Care*. Mosby, London.

29 Campbell AV (1984) *Moderated Love, A Theology of Professional Care*. SPCK, London.

30 Morse J, Bottorff J, Andreson G *et al.* (1992) Beyond empathy: expanding expressions of caring. *Journal of Advanced Nursing*. **17**: 809–21.

31 Van Amburg R (1996) A Copernican revolution in clinical ethics: engagement versus disengagement. *The American Journal of Occupational Therapy*. **51**(3): 186–90.

32 Cassell EJ (1999) Diagnosing suffering: a perspective. *Annals of Internal Medicine*. **131**(7): 531–4.
33 James N (1989) Emotional labour: skill and work in social regulation of feelings. *Sociological Review*. **37**(1): 15–42.
34 Ross LA (1994) Spiritual aspects of nursing. *Journal of Advanced Nursing*. **19**: 439–47.
35 Wilkinson K (1996) The concept of hope in life-threatening illness. *Palliative Care*. **11**(10): 659–61.
36 MacLeod R, Carter H (1999) Health professionals' perception of hope: understanding its significance in the care of people who are dying. *Mortality*. **4**(3): 309–17.
37 Dawson PJ (1997) A reply to Goddard's 'spirituality as integrative energy'. *Journal of Advanced Nursing*. **25**(2): 282–9.
38 Stanworth R (2004) *Recognizing Spiritual Needs in People Who Are Dying*. Oxford University Press, Oxford.
39 Larner G (1998) Through a glass darkly. *Theory and Psychology*. **8**(4): 549–72.
40 Becker B (1999) Narratives of pain in later life and conventions of storytelling. *Journal of Aging Studies*. **13**(1): 73–87.
41 Gee JP (1991) A linguistic approach to narrative. *Journal of Narrative and Life History*. **1**: 15–39.
42 King G (2004) The meaning of life experiences: application of a meta-model to rehabilitation sciences and services. *American Journal of Orthopsychiatry*. **74**(1): 72–88.
43 Culliford L (2002) Spirituality and clinical care: spiritual values and skills are increasingly recognised as necessary aspects of clinical care. *BMJ*. **325**(7378): 1434–5.
44 Kliewer S (2004) Allowing spirituality into the healing process. *The Journal of Family Practice*. **53**(8): 616–24.
45 McColl AM (2000) Spirit, occupation and disability. *Canadian Journal of Occupational Therapy*. **67**(4): 217–28.
46 Mayers CA (2004) Towards understanding spirituality. *British Journal of Occupational Therapy*. **67**(5): 191.
47 Whalley Hammell K (2001) Intrinsicality: reconsidering spirituality, meaning(s) and mandates. *Canadian Journal of Occupational Therapy*. **68**(3): 186–94.
48 Dyson J, Cobb M, Forman D (1997) The meaning of spirituality: a literature review. *Journal of Advanced Nursing*. **26**: 1183–8.
49 McEwan W (2004) Spirituality in nursing, what are the issues? *Orthopaedic Nursing*. **23**(5): 321–6.
50 Draper P, McSherry W (2002) A critical view of spirituality and spiritual assessment. *Journal of Advanced Nursing*. **39**(1): 1–2.
51 Sermabeikian P (1994) Our clients, ourselves: the spiritual perspective and social work practice. *Social Work*. **39**(2): 178–83.
52 Walter T (2002) Spirituality in palliative care: opportunity or burden? *Palliative Medicine*. **16**: 133–9.
53 Daaleman TP (2004) Religion, spirituality, and the practice of medicine. *Journal of the American Board of Family Practice*. **17**: 370–6.
54 Newman M (1997) Experiencing the whole. *Advances in Nursing Science*. **20**(1): 34–9.
55 McSherry W, Ross L (2002) Dilemmas of spiritual assessment: considerations for nursing practice. *Journal of Advanced Nursing*. **38**(5): 479–88.
56 Farvis RA (2005) Ethical considerations in spiritual care. *International Journal of Palliative Nursing*. **11**(4): 189.
57 Walter T (1994) *The Revival of Death*. Routledge, London.
58 Collins JS, Paul S, West-Frasier J (2001) The utilization of spirituality in occupational therapy: beliefs, practices, and perceived barriers. *Occupational Therapy in Health Care*. **14**(3/4): 73–92.
59 Callister LC, Matsumura G (2004) Threading spirituality throughout nursing education. *Holistic Nursing Practice*. **May/June**: 160–6.
60 McCord G, Gilchrist J, Grossman SD *et al*. (2004) Discussing spirituality with patients: a rational and ethical approach. *Annals of Family Medicine*. **2**. 356–61.
61 Harrison J, Burnard P (1993) *Spirituality and Nursing Practice*. Avenbury, Aldershot.
62 McSherry W (2000) Education issues surrounding the teaching of spirituality. *Nursing Standard*. **14**(42): 40–3.

CHAPTER 5

Sustaining hope

Wendy Greenstreet and Mo Fiddian

Introduction

Desroche[1] compares hope to a rope that in myth is thrown in the air, anchored in cloud and carries the weight of the man who climbs it. Such is the nature of hope, remaining intangible and eluding explanation in an era of scientific reason, and yet clung to in life's most difficult moments. This chapter will explore the concept of hope, initially by reviewing its status as an aspect of spirituality, and then the role of theory in attempting to describe what constitutes hope. Culture and religiosity are discussed in relation to their significance in determining the lived experience of hope. Hopelessness, its causes and the implications for health and social care professionals are considered. Finally, studies that suggest ways in which hope can be maintained and inspired in the recipients of health and social care are interpreted for use in practice.

Hope as an aspect of spirituality

In situating hope within the concept of spirituality, it is not only a theme of spiritual need in itself but constitutes a part of each of the themes of meaning, relationship and forgiveness. It might be that the object of hope is meaningful to the individual,[2] but a more dominant component of hope is the personal dimension or spirit of hope that revolves around a core theme of meaning, associated with a sense of the possible or feeling of empowerment.[3] Theory explaining the concept of hope regularly makes reference to the importance and role of relationship regarding hope,[4-6] not only with significant others but also with the self. It is perhaps the ability of the self to transcend the challenges faced in health and social care that best describes hope. This is clearly expressed by Bauckham and Hart:[7]

> Hope ... is a vital function of imagination lying at the heart of our humanity. Specifically, it is the capacity to imagine otherwise, to transcend the boundaries of the present in a quest for something more, something better, than the present affords. (p.72)

Forgiveness can be the object of hope in situations imbued with guilt.

Theoretical exploration of what constitutes hope

Theoretical analysis of definitions and conceptual usage have identified various attributes of hope.[4-6,8] The key elements of definitions in published literature, including research studies, are summarised by Cutcliffe and Herth.[9] Common themes are that hope is individualised, is dynamic and future oriented. These elements illustrate both the temporal and contextual nature of hope, both of which are significant in the delivery of care. Future orientation is related to the individual's past as well as their present circumstances and can be illustrated by considering a lifespan perspective.

Carson[10] refers to Erikson's (1963) work describing hope as the outcome of the first developmental task in life borne out of the balance achieved between trust and mistrust. In trusting their mothers, infants begin to hope, to anticipate the future and hope that their needs will be met and comfort given. The individual variation that would result in this development supports Snyder *et al.*'s[11] view that hope is individually variable, but an enduring disposition, an aptitude that is transferable to different contexts. This is reflected in individual difference in degrees of hope. Individuals reporting higher levels of hope do not perceive their goals as more difficult, but as challenges with potential for success, or within the context of health and social care they would exhibit less distress than those with low levels of hope. On reaching mid-life, MacKinlay[12] suggests that hope is present in activity, in doing, through meaning found in work, parenting and other activities. This view contrasts with ageing, in that, generally, post-mid-life hope is associated more with transcendence, a deepening sense of interiority and a transition from an emphasis on doing to a greater focus on being.

The identification and understanding of different components of hope can facilitate health and social care professionals' ability to assess need of hope-enhancing strategies by those in their care. However, hope is a complex construct.[3] It is primarily an experience of wholeness. The intangible qualities of hope are lost in theory that reduces hope to a uni-dimensional framework or merely a list of attributes, elements or characteristics. Multiplicity of focus is reflected even in its grammatical use both as a noun, concerned with a feeling of expectation or desire, a person or thing that gives cause for hope or grounds for hoping, and as a verb, to expect and desire, to intend, if possible, to do something.[13]

A model of hope that emanated from a study by Dufault and Martocchio[14] defined hope as both dynamic and multidimensional. Although critical of the study's failure to describe aspects of the research process, Cutcliffe and Herth[9] own that this study does provide thought-provoking propositions regarding the spheres and dimensions of hope. Hope is described as constituting two spheres, generalised and particularised hope, which have six psychosocial dimensions (Box 5.1).

Box 5.1 The six psychosocial dimensions of generalised and particularised hope[14]

1   Affective: sensations and emotions that are part of the hoping process
2   Cognitive: e.g. wishing, imagining, interpreting and judging in relation to hope
3   Behavioural: action orientation in relation to hope
4   Affiliative: individual's relatedness beyond self with others, nature and 'God' or higher power
5   Temporal: individual's experience of time; past, present and future
6   Contextual: life situations that surround, influence and are part of individual's hope

---

Generalised hope 'protects against despair when a person is deprived of particular hopes'[14] (p.380). It is concerned with 'being' and is a rather nebulous, personal dimension[15] that provides a sense of something beneficial to come, a positive glow, a global rather than focused component that provides motivation to carry on with life,[16] a way of living in hope.[17] It is an important aspect of hope to nurture in those whose circumstances or ill health mean that 'being' rather than 'doing' is more uplifting, for example for those with advanced chronic disease or who are dying.

Particularised hope, however, is concerned with 'doing', involves activity and is focused on a particular goal.[15] It reflects the expectation that what exists in the present time can be improved upon. Hence for those in health and social care, their goal(s) may drive those activities that move the individual towards hope of wellbeing, cure or better social circumstances. Particularised hope provides an incentive for constructive coping and devising of options to realise goals.[16]

These descriptions promote a better understanding of hope, but it is important not to lose sight of hope as a holistic concept. Individuals would experience both generalised and particularised hope, although the dominance of each sphere may vary over time. Benzein *et al.*[17] use recollection to describe the duality of this unity as the lived experience of hope (Figure 5.1).

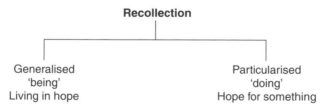

Recollection

Generalised	Particularised
'being'	'doing'
Living in hope	Hope for something

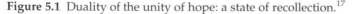

Figure 5.1 Duality of the unity of hope: a state of recollection.[17]

Merton[18] gives a more contemplative description of recollection as:

> ...a change of spiritual focus and an attuning of our whole soul to what is beyond and above ourselves ... a simplification of our state of mind and our spiritual activity... The spirit that is recollected is quiet and detached, at

least at its depths... Recollection is more than a mere turning inward upon ourselves... Sometimes we are more recollected, quieter ... when we see *through* exterior things ... it does not deny sensible things, it sets them in order... Recollection should not be seen as an absence, but as a presence. It makes us, first of all, present to ourselves. It makes us present to whatever reality is most significant in the moment of time in which we are living. (pp.191–2)

In a study to identify a structure for hope based on personal meaning, Nekolaichuk *et al.*[3] used the six social and psychological dimensions included in Dufault and Martocchio's[14] model of hope (*see* Box 5.1) as an initial framework of content to develop a connotative structure reflecting the feeling invoked by the term 'hope' rather than just its meaning. In this way, they claim to capture the qualitative experience of hope. This new model identifies three interconnected factors (Figure 5.2) that blend 'doing' and 'being' as constituents of hope.[15] The first and most dominant dimension is that of personal spirit, which incorporates a core theme of meaning. This dimension includes a prominent evaluative component in its association with what is of value, which is complemented by a subjective component that includes, for example, caring. The second dimension is that of risk, a situational dimension that emphasises balance between uncertainty and predictability. Stability and expectation as part of predictability are underpinned by an important theme of boldness in feeling confident. Lastly, authentic caring constitutes an interpersonal dimension that blends the credibility of hope and comfort. This model provides a greater understanding of the unique, person-centred experience of hope.

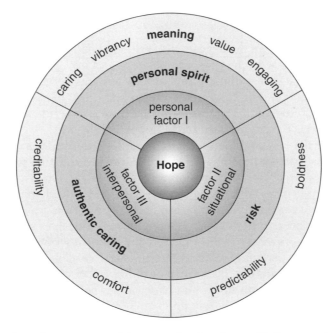

Figure 5.2 The three interconnected factors reflecting the qualitative meaning of hope.[3]

Culture and the lived experience of hope

Cultural affiliation influences people's understanding of hope, and therefore this concept should be viewed in its social context.[19] Secularism is a belief system that is associated with Western culture. It is concerned with a reliance on an individual's reason in all matters and divides the sacred from the secular. Reason is therefore a source of coping in situations of threat that motivate hope. There is a tendency to assume that secularism is automatically in conflict with religion, and this is not surprising given that it engenders an agnostic reservation of judgement in all matters that lie outside of reason, and so would treat the sacred with suspicion.[20]

Religion dominates or underpins most societies and therefore impacts the experience of hope and its ultimate goals. 'Religiosity' is a term used to describe how people express their religious beliefs and practices and the importance given to them.[21]

In a study by Benzein et al.[19] of hope in healthy Swedish Christians (Pentecostalists), hope was experienced primarily as future imagined reality of God's promise of reunion with mankind in eternity, but faith was so integrated into their lives that hope was also a present transcendent reality, 'life as a walk with God, who is always present' (p.1065). A third, but less significant source of hope, was short-sighted personal goals built on weak feelings and linked to the possibility of being disappointed, for example in finding a partner or achieving self-fulfilment. Holt's study[22] of Hispanic cultural interpretation of hope in a rural Dominican village found that the life of this social group was rooted in Christian religion (Roman Catholicism) with faith in God as the primary source of hope:

> Hope is an essential but dynamic life force that grows out of faith in God, is supported by relationships, resources and work, and results in energy necessary to work for a desired future. (p.1116)

These studies exemplify an intrinsic form of religiosity. Religion is taken seriously, and faith provides hope in the present, the 'here and now', through the sense of communion with God in religious practice that is incorporated in daily life.[21] Future hope is motivated by faith in the imagined reality of eternity. The studies illustrate that even in different cultures, for those who are intrinsically religious, faith in their God is the primary source of hope in their lives.

In comparing the Hispanic definition of hope with definitions developed from studies of mainstream populations in the US, Holt[22] found that when faith as an attribute of hope was included in definitions given by American mainstream groups, it was given equal rather than primary status and that the American definitions did not support the emphasis on hope as essential in life, or work as an important way to sustain hope. This demonstrates differences in cultural experience of hope. Those Americans who included faith as an attribute of hope but not its primary source may use religion as an instrument, that is motivated by extrinsic religiosity where religious practices are important for sociability, security, status or solace.[21] The religious community may well be a resource for support in maintaining hope for the extrinsically religious.

Eastern culture based on Hindu and Buddhist faiths focus on the concept of karma rather than hope (Burkhard Scherer, personal communication, 2005). In a study situated in rural Eastern culture, Tongprateep[23] described the essential elements of spirituality among Thai elders. The participants were Buddhists and believed in the law of karma; that good or evil actions bring about effects not only in the present life but also in the next. So for the Thai elders, hope centred on an accumulation of meritorious acts resulting in good effect in this life and the next. The main objective of merit making was to eliminate selfishness and greed, to 'purify myself ... develop peace of mind' (p.200). The reality of life under the law of karma helped the elders remain calm when faced with difficulties:

> I have confidence in my life that I have done good deeds. It makes me have a peaceful mind when I think about my past meritorious actions. (p.212)

Happiness, suffering and illness were all considered karmic results. Meditation was considered a way of making merit and proved beneficial in enhancing self-awareness, developing a peaceful mind, improving sleep, releasing stress and anxiety, and enhancing physical health. All the participants had become more interested in their religion as they grew older. As time had passed, the elders had experienced negative and positive life events that had helped them more fully understand the law of karma and other Buddhist doctrine. The more they understood, the better they were able to practise in their daily lives. This suggests that age moved Thai elders towards an increasing intrinsic religiosity.

It is important for professionals to be aware of the potential shared and different sources and meanings of hope in the cultural and religious groups represented by the clients or patients in their care. Western, secularised culture values control[24] and so may be predisposed to a stronger focus on particularised hope utilising information, medicine and technology to achieve their goals, whereas rural Eastern culture exemplified by Tongprateep's[23] study may be more prone to focus on generalised hope, concerned with 'being' in the moment, using meditation to release stress and anxiety, and reflecting on investment in past activity as a source of experience and confidence in facing the difficult circumstances they find themselves in.

Control of information in different cultures can empower patients and clients to make choices in setting goals to maintain hope or protect them from being informed of the details of their situation to avoid the loss of hope. Western culture promotes individual determination to be an ideal. Patients are informed of their situation based on the right to autonomy, whereas in Eastern Thai culture there is an adherence to truth telling grounded in veracity. However, some cultures support non-disclosure to patients to protect them from loss of hope and serenity as the social norm, and therefore relatives are expected to protect those who are ill or distressed. Examples of cultures that practise non-disclosure of a diagnosis of cancer include Italian, and Americans of Hispanic and Asian background.[25]

Potential loss of hope

Although areas of hopelessness are inherent in humanity,[26] the individual suffering that results in the loss of all hope comes from relational difficulties and social adversity.[27] The loss of hope then can be cumulative rather than incidental. Those hoping for cure, for example, may be aware of disease progression and loss of normality of social role, as well as the presence of tension in significant relationships as independence ebbs away, long before any formal announcement of treatment failure. The very style of conveying information can result in further loss of hope if an individual is given a sense of being 'written off'.[28] Also, professional carers have been found to associate hope with an absence of disease or a lack of disease progression and so have been less able to convey hope in the care of those with extremely disabling disorders.[15] Dissonance can occur between the professional's knowledge and the patient's perception of the situation. Patients might use hope in being 'unrealistically realistic' as an attempt to cope with what might otherwise appear hopeless.[29] Quality of life has been described as the difference or gap between an individual's expectations and their experiences of reality.[30] A good quality of life occurs when hope matches expectations or experience. Paradoxically, when a goal that constitutes an expectation central to quality of life is severely threatened, the hopeful patient may expend a large amount of energy fiercely defending that hope.[31]

Hope work is accomplished through conversation. In situations where hope work is focused on cure, related to getting better, or on palliative care, concerned with feeling better, interactions seem to be more common between professionals and patients rather than among professional carers. However, in work for dismantling hope of cure, when nothing more can prevent the patient from dying, interaction shifts to being more typically among professional carers. When curative hope is dismantled, palliative hope needs to be maintained.[32] Therefore, an important issue that health and social care professionals need to be aware of is that the nature of their discussions with patients or clients, their use of interpersonal skills, their ability to 'be with' the patient, are potential resources that will contribute to those in their care maintaining, finding or losing hope. Post-White et al.[33] found that hope was highly correlated with a sense of coherence. Finding meaning and making sense of a situation are important aspects of hope and coherence, but identifying and mobilising resources are equally significant. Professional carers need to encourage or facilitate the means for their patients or clients to maintain or find hope and coherence.

Assessment of hopefulness

Hope is a dynamic process so assessment needs to be brief and repeated as often as required.[34] The intangible essence of hope makes a qualitative approach to assessment the most appropriate, centred on a rapport that facilitates a trusting relationship. Tools that measure hope are of little value in clinical contexts because of their length and complexity,[5,35,36] but they do provide useful guides for those wanting or needing practice in framing relevant questions to include in conversations that assess hopefulness in patients as they deliver treatment and/or care. Penfold and Morse[34] point out that assessment needs to address the course of hope, including the fluctuations in hopefulness, commonly encountered by patients or clients developing or sustaining hope. Observation of actions that allow some relief from the work of hope when energy is depleted are important, and not to be confused with a state of hopelessness. Relief may be sought in beneficial activity such as meditation and relaxation or through potentially damaging behaviours such as ingestion of alcohol or overeating.

Hope is also a multidimensional concept and this needs to be reflected in the assessment and provision of care. Dufault and Martocchio's[14] description of particularised and generalised spheres of hope provide a means of framing different approaches when considering the importance of this concept in care environments. Particularised hope would therefore need to be nurtured in situations that would benefit from goal-oriented activity where 'doing' was considered beneficial, and similarly, generalised hope nurtured in circumstances where an increased focus on 'being' more appropriate, depending on the situation, as well as on cultural and religious beliefs. This is not to suggest that a patient's hope will not constitute both particularised and generalised spheres at any one time but that the emphasis on sourcing hope might shift.

Promoting goal-oriented 'doing' to enhance hope

Using advanced techniques of concept analysis, Morse and Doberneck[37] identified seven abstract and universal components in the process of developing hope (Box 5.2).

Box 5.2   The process of developing hope: seven abstract and universal components[36]

1   Realistic initial assessment of the predicament or threat
2   Envisioning alternatives and setting goals
3   Bracing for negative outcomes
4   Realistic assessment of personal and external resources
5   Solicitation of mutually supportive relationships
6   Continuous evaluation for signs that reinforce selected goals
7   A determination to endure

In comparing the manifestations of these components in four groups of patients/ clients (those undergoing heart surgery, with spinal cord injury, having survived breast cancer and breastfeeding mothers returning to work), they found that in each group the seven universal abstract properties were identified to achieve different patterns of hope. The outcome of the study was a markedly goal-oriented description of the concept of hope:

> Hope is a response to a threat that results in the setting of a desired goal; the awareness of the cost of not achieving the goal; the planning to make the goal a reality; the assessment, selection, and use of all internal and external resources and supports that will assist in achieving the goal; and the re-evaluation and revision of the plan while enduring, working, and striving to reach the desired goal. (p.284)

This view of hope as a process offers a means of assessing and guiding the support offered to each patient or client who is particularly focused on activity-based goal setting to achieve hope of future improvement of their current circumstances. The assessment of hope in stages facilitates 'stage-specific strategies to augment the development of hopefulness'[34] (p.1060) specific to individual need. This does not mean that hope is a linear process of prescribed stages but fluid, in that individuals 'may cycle in and out of stages until they are ready to move on'[34] (p.1060).

Regardless of the situation, when individuals assess the predicament they find themselves in, it is the degree of threat to personal safety that is the primary factor that contributes to the intensity of hope. This intensity serves as a motivating force. It is important for professional carers not to make assumptions about what determines intensity of personal threat. For example, they may consider that the intensity of hoping for a heart transplant and hoping for breastfeeding to continue would differ, but Morse and Doberneck[37] found that both goals 'appeared important to the people concerned and occupied much of their time and energy' (p.283).

This initial assessment is not usually a single event, and on occasions denial may be used to escape from the reality of the situation. Realistic assessment is usually 'pieced together' and so professionals need to be careful in pitching the level and amount of information given to facilitate 'fitting the pieces together' and avoid overwhelming the patient or client. Key information needs to be repeated and questioning encouraged. Active listening is important as patients or clients reiterate the circumstances of their predicament in an attempt to make sense of reality.[34]

Realistic assessment includes envisioning alternative goals and bracing for negative outcomes. Fear of negative outcome was found to be a motivating force for individual action that makes hope powerful.[37] Therefore, health and social care professionals need to support those who express fear, rather than deny that negative outcomes are a possibility. The choice of goal must be attractive or desired[14] and so must be the patient's or client's choice. Professional expertise is important in moulding formulation of goals[34] but should not be prescriptive. For those immobilised by hopelessness, with negative outcomes seen as inevitable rather than possible, resulting in an inability to set a goal, the professional carer must acknowledge areas of bona fide hopelessness but also identify and encourage awareness of hopeful aspects of the situation.[26]

Morse and Doberneck[37] found that it was not until after the individual had tentatively selected a goal and assessed what they had to lose that they assessed their personal ability to achieve the goal(s) and the availability of other resources that would help. Again, this was a realistic assessment with individuals very aware of possible negative outcomes and so not wanting to set themselves up to fail. If the plan for goal attainment was not found to be feasible at this stage, a new goal or set of goals were chosen and the process repeated.

The attainment of a goal is not achieved alone, but includes the solicitation of mutually supportive relationships. These relationships are balanced and so it is rare for all members to have doubts about the feasibility of a goal at the same time. Support strategies used in these relationships may be 'hands-on' support or indirect support that bolsters the individual's ability to deal with their situation, for example, affirming personal attributes such as courage or endurance.[34] Professional carers may well be party to these mutually supportive relationships.

Between selecting and attaining goal(s) the individual may search for some indication that they had made the right choice. Evidence that this is the case is essential if hope is to be maintained. Professionals can facilitate discussion of how patients perceive their progress.[34] Multiple goals may increase the need to revise the means or actions to attain goals. Health and social care professionals may contribute to honest appraisal of progress that strengthens hope. They can also offer support should feedback identify the need for revision of plans to achieve goals or, if necessary, help in changing goals so that they are attainable. The length of time between setting goals and their achievement has to be endured. This endurance demands energy. Personal and professional carers can all contribute in encouraging the individual in their determination to persevere.

Case study illustrating process and the seven components of hope

John was 19 years old and had suffered a traumatic through knee amputation of his left lower leg in a motorcycle accident. His youth and robust physical health contributed to his surviving physiological shock. Both his recovery from the surgery necessary for formation of his stump and the healing of the stump wound were uncomplicated.

From the outset John conveyed a stoic disposition, assessing his predicament as one of relative 'luck' because he had lost his leg and not his life. The intensity of his motivation to achieve his goal of a return to as near normal mobility as possible was driven by his desire for employment, to sustain relationships as he had known them and recapture his image of self (component 1).

He 'pieced together' information from professional carers. Nursing and medical staff outlined a timetable and order of goals, from stump wound healing to use of a temporary prosthetic limb and ultimately his own prosthesis. Alongside this, physiotherapists explained how he would be helped to move on from transferring to a wheelchair, to use of crutches and then to learning a new style of walking using his prosthesis. This information guided his intent in negotiating intermediate goals (component 2).

Phantom sensations 'felt' in his missing limb, a common occurrence following amputation, challenged his sense of reality and his morale. In conversation, he seemed to be bracing himself for some negative outcomes, possibly less choice in relation to employment and a potential need to review his usual activities with friends (component 3).

John drove himself to meet his goals, encouraged by positive feedback from staff, friends and family (component 5), as well as by his own self-assessment of progress (component 4). However, he did need to re-evaluate his goals and personal resources when he overstretched himself and fell. His morale was badly shaken by this event, but it was an opportunity for both professional carers and family to encourage him to review his plans, not in outcome, but in the time schedule he had set himself (component 6). He was encouraged to nurture himself a little to sustain the energy needed to endure the challenges he faced (component 7).

Promoting 'being' to enhance hope

Generalised hope is concerned with 'being', a way of living in hope.[17] It is an important aspect of hope to nurture in those patients or clients whose circumstances are chronic or life limiting, where the focus is perhaps more on hope in the 'here and now'. Hope as a way of 'being' is concerned with shifting perception rather than goal-focused action. Future aims may be concerned with quality of life rather than goal-focused achievement.

In a study exploring the meaning of hope in terminally ill adults, Herth[38] identified strategies that are used to foster hope (Box 5.3). These strategies are a potentially useful guide in maintaining and inspiring generalised hope in those needing to focus particularly on 'being' in the present moment, and are therefore applicable in a range of health and social care settings. The strategies work on the premise that giving up on particular hopes does not mean giving up on hope altogether.

Box 5.3   Seven hope-fostering strategies[38,39]

1   Interpersonal connectedness
2   Attainable aims
3   Spiritual base
4   Uplifting memories
5   Affirmation of worth
6   Personal attributes
7   Lightheartedness

Interpersonal connectedness is described by Buckley and Herth[39] as comprising meaningful relationships and being loved and giving love. In health and social care contexts, professional carers figure alongside family and friends in constituting significant relationships with clients/patients. Acknowledging the universal nature of hope may be the first step in enabling professional carers to make interpersonal connections with those in their care. Having a sense of something that is important to all humanity could provide some common ground on which to start building a therapeutic relationship. Professionals can then enable clients/patients to retain important attachments such as family relationships and personal friendships.

Attainable aims are related to setting goals and maintaining independence. In this way, generalised hope does not exclude goal setting but acknowledges a shifting rather than focused goal. For example, clients/patients may wish to shift the focus of future hopes from themselves to hopes for their family and friends. They can therefore still imagine a future and make plans and decisions in regard to that future. Independence is maintained by allowing opportunities for clients/patients to manage their affairs in their own way.

An understanding of a client/patient's spiritual base requires an understanding of their spirituality, so that professional carers can facilitate opportunity for expression and practices associated with their source of faith. This may be religious practice, having the opportunity to listen to music that holds particular meaning or some may choose moments of solitude.

Uplifting memories have a temporal dimension, in that the client/patient's past is reflected on in the present and contributes to hope and its association with the future. Relationships that are open to sharing these moments of reflection provide opportunities to affirm worth in the expression of love and appreciation by friends and family.

Similarly, personal attributes or characteristics, such as optimism and cheerfulness, if nurtured provide opportunity for lightheartedness. Spontaneity, sensitivity in the use of humour and the ability to laugh as the moment dictates creates joy that contributes to sustaining hope.

Case study illustrating seven hope-fostering strategies

After successful symptom control, Rosemary, a 72-year-old lady, was being prepared for discharge from hospice. A sprightly woman who greatly valued her independence, she was pleased to be returning to her own home.

Rosemary had a good rapport with a number of the hospice staff and also a close, supportive relationship with her daughter. Professional carers were skilled in enabling her relationship with her daughter to continue as normal and so reflect their mutual affection (strategy 1). Rosemary had attained the aims that she had hoped for. Her symptoms were sufficiently managed to enable her to make the choice to return home and spend what time she had left with her daughter (strategy 2).

During her stay, Rosemary drew strength from the sight of a magnificent, old, gnarled tree that was growing outside the window of her room. She used the tree to help her make sense of her experience of the process of dying. The tree's firm roots represented an established history and her legacy to and in her daughter. Its flourishing symbolised that life would go on (strategy 3). A member of the caring team provided Rosemary with a photograph of the tree that would provide a source of uplifting moments on return home (strategy 4). This demonstrated sensitivity to Rosemary's attachment to this tree and was an affirmation of her worth as a person (strategy 5).

Her engaging nature reflected personal attributes that facilitated lighthearted conversation despite her deteriorating health (strategies 6 and 7).

Conclusion

Hope is an integral part of the concept of spirituality and interwoven within all themes of spiritual need. Although a number of definitions have been referred to throughout the course of this chapter, no one definition is offered as reflecting the gestalt, wholeness of this concept. Instead an attempt has been made to describe comprehensively the multidimensional nature and meaning of hope. Culture and religiosity are included as essential parts of shaping and determining the meaning of hope for individuals, as well as their choice and means of sustaining hope. Assessment of hopefulness for those in health and social care needs to be qualitative, elicited within an established relationship with the carer. Suggestions for professionals to support and facilitate both problem-focused action and emotion-focused adjustment of perception[40] to sustain hope for those who are particularly focused on 'doing' or those who are generally concerned with 'being' are made. Hope cannot be given, it can only be maintained or inspired. Health and social care professionals need to be aware of their influence on patients' and clients' hopefulness or loss of hope.

References

1 Desroche H (1979) *The Sociology of Hope*. Routledge and Kegan Paul, London.
2 Frankl V (1984) *Man's Search for Meaning*. Washington Square Press, New York, NY.
3 Nekolaichuk CL, Jevne RF, Maguire TO (1999) Structuring the meaning of hope in health and illness. *Social Science and Medicine*. **48**: 591–605.
4 Stephenson C (1991) The concept of hope revisited for nursing. *Journal of Advanced Nursing*. **16**: 1456–61.
5 Farran JC, Wilken C, Popovich JM (1992) Clinical assessment of hope. *Issues in Mental Health Nursing*. **13**: 129–38.
6 Kylma J, Vehvilainen-Julkunen K (1997) Hope in nursing research: a meta-analysis of the ontological and epistemological foundations of research on hope. *Journal of Advanced Nursing*. **25**(2): 364–71.
7 Bauckham R, Hart T (1999) *Hope Against Hope*. Darton, Longman and Todd, London.
8 Benzein E, Saveman B (1998) Nurses' perception of hope in patients with cancer: a palliative care perspective. *Cancer Nursing*. **21**(1): 10–16.
9 Cutcliffe JR, Herth KA (2002) The concept of hope in nursing 1: its origins, background and nature. *British Journal of Nursing*. **11**(12): 832–40.
10 Carson VB (1989) *Spiritual Dimensions of Nursing Practice*. Saunders, Philadelphia, PA.
11 Snyder CR, Harris C, Anderson JR *et al.* (1991) The will and the ways: development and validation of an individual-differences measure of hope. *Journal of Personality and Social Psychology*. **60**(4): 570–85.
12 MacKinlay E (2001) *The Spiritual Dimension of Ageing*. Jessica Kingsley, London.
13 Pearsall J (ed.) (2001) *The Concise Oxford Dictionary* (10e). Oxford University Press, Oxford.
14 Dufault K, Martocchio B (1985) Hope: its spheres and dimensions. *Nursing Clinics of North America*. **20**: 379–91.
15 MacLeod R, Carter H (1999) Health professionals' perception of hope: understanding its significance in the care of people who are dying. *Mortality*. **4**(3): 309–17.
16 Cutcliffe JR, Herth KA (2002) The concept of hope in nursing 4: hope and gerontological nursing. *British Journal of Nursing*. **11**(17): 1148–56.
17 Benzein E, Norberg A, Saveman B (2001) The meaning of the lived experience of hope in patients with cancer in palliative home care. *Palliative Medicine*. **15**(2): 117–26.
18 Merton T (1955) *No Man is an Island*. Hollis and Carter, London.
19 Benzein E, Norberg A, Saveman B (1998) Hope: future imagined reality. The meaning of hope as described by a group of healthy Pentecostalists. *Journal of Advanced Nursing*. **28**(5): 1063–70
20 Parkes CM, Laungani P, Young B (eds) (1997) *Death and Bereavement Across Cultures*. Routledge, London.
21 Fehring RJ, Miller JF, Shaw C (1997) Spiritual well-being, religiosity, hope, depression, and other mood states in elderly people coping with cancer. *Oncology Nursing Forum*. **24**(4): 663–71.
22 Holt J (2000) Exploration of the concept of hope in the Dominican Republic. *Journal of Advanced Nursing*. **32**(5): 1116–25.
23 Tongprateep T (2000) The essential elements of spirituality among Thai elders. *Journal of Advanced Nursing*. **31**(1): 197–203.
24 Friedemann M, Mouch J, Racey T (2002) Nursing the spirit: the Framework of Systemic Organization. *Journal of Advanced Nursing*. **39**(4): 325–32.
25 Berger J (1998) Culture and ethnicity in clinical care. *Archives of Internal Medicine*. **158**(19): 2085–90.
26 McGee R (1984) Hope: a factor influencing crisis resolution. *Advances in Nursing Science*. **July**: 34–44.
27 Aldridge D (2003) *Suicide, The Tragedy of Hopelessness*. Jessica Kingsley, London.
28 Flemming K (1997) The meaning of hope to palliative care patients. *International Journal of Palliative Nursing*. **3**(1): 14–18.
29 Wilkinson K (1996) The concept of hope in life-threatening illness. *Palliative Care*. **11**(10): 659–61.

30 Calman KC (1984) Quality of life in cancer patients: an hypothesis. *Journal of Medical Ethics.* **10**(3): 124–7.

31 Penson J (2000) A hope is not a promise: fostering hope within palliative care. *International Journal of Palliative Nursing.* **6**(2): 94–8.

32 Perakyla A (1991) Hope work in the care of seriously ill patients. *Qualitative Health Research.* **1**(4): 407–33.

33 Post-White J, Ceronsky C, Kreitzer M *et al.* (1996) Hope, spirituality, sense of coherence, and quality of life in patients with cancer. *Oncology Nursing Forum.* **23**(10): 1571–9.

34 Penfold J, Morse J (1997) Strategies for assessing and fostering hope: the Hope Assessment Guide. *Oncology Nursing Forum.* **24**(6): 1055–63.

35 Herth KA (1991) Development and refinement of an instrument to measure hope. *Scholarly Inquiry for Nursing Practice.* **5**(1): 39–51.

36 Herth KA (1992) An abbreviated instrument to measure hope: development and psychometric evaluation. *Journal of Advanced Nursing.* **17**: 1251–9.

37 Morse JM, Doberneck B (1995) Delineating the concept of hope. *Image-Journal of Nursing Scholarship.* **27**(4): 277–85.

38 Herth K (1990) Fostering hope in terminally ill people. *Journal of Advanced Nursing.* **15**: 1250–9.

39 Buckley J, Herth K (2004) Fostering hope in terminally ill patients. *Nursing Standard.* **19**(10): 33–41.

40 Chaplin J, McIntyre R (2001) Hope: an exploration of selected literature. In: Kinghorn S, Gamlin R (eds) *Palliative Nursing, Bringing Comfort and Hope.* Baillière Tindall, Edinburgh.

CHAPTER 6

Soul works: the relevance of spirituality to a healthy workplace

Stephen G Wright

Every creature strives, by its activity, to communicate its own perfect being, in its own fashion, to another; and in this it tends toward an imitation of the divine causality.

Thomas Aquinas[1] (p.256)

Unholy work?

It was close to the end of a challenging conference on the theme of 'spirituality and health'. It was one of the first, if not *the* first, on this subject in the UK some 15 years ago, and 200 delegates had gathered at the magnificent Bishop's Palace in Durham. Under the shadow of its awesome cathedral, the conference retired to the debating hall to explore the relevance of spirituality to the workplace. The debate lurched from view to view as delegates related their experiences. But it was the tearful voice of one woman, an occupational therapist as I recall, whose voice and words remain with me still.

> 'It has been wonderful to be here,' she said, 'to be among people who think and feel the same as me, to realise that I'm not on my own in this, but how can I go back to work when my heart and soul are not welcome there?'

That phrase 'heart and soul not welcome' seems to echo the common experience of so many people in the workplace. For many people, work has become not a source of joy, meaning, purpose and connection (the very stuff of spirituality), but of disconnection, meaninglessness and alienation.[2–5] Healthy workplaces embrace (encouraged or indeed forced by legislation) attention to the social, physical and psychological wellbeing of workers. The concepts of holism – that everything is connected, is part of 'all that is' and nothing is truly separate – have entered the jargon of much of modern Western health and social care and business. Although holism has become much debased in its meaning in common parlance, one impact of embracing this paradigm into the workplace has been to place increasing emphasis on a hitherto largely ignored aspect of what it is to be human – spirituality. If laws and conventions require employers to pay attention, for example to the physical welfare of their staff, can this same welfare be expected to attend to their spiritual wellbeing as well?

For the purposes of this chapter I make a distinction between religion and spirituality, although the two are closely related and overlap. Everybody seeks meaning, purpose, direction and connection in life. We all at some point ask questions of what it's all about and why we are here, seeking answers to all those great existential questions like 'Who am I?', 'Why am I here?', 'Where am I going?' and 'How do I get there?'. We all pursue relationships, work and activities that nurture and feel 'right' to us. For some people this pursuit is essentially God-centred, embracing the belief in some divine being(s). For others, it is essentially atheistic or at least agnostic, such as humanism or Buddhism. Our spirituality is therefore the very roots of our being – who we think we are, why we are here and what we should do with our lives. Religion can be seen as the ritual, liturgy, dogma and the various practices that we collectively bring to our spiritual life to codify and unify it with others. Indeed some, if not most, religions provide ready-made answers to those questions we ask about the nature of our being and purpose. Religion provides a channel for the expression of our spirituality. Thus, everybody is spiritual but not everybody is religious. We all seek meaning, purpose, relationship and connectedness in life, but not everybody chooses to channel that quest through the more formal structure and belief system of a religion.

Religiosity and spirituality are profoundly influenced by the familial, social and cultural circumstances in which we live and grow. Recent studies suggest that we are prone to the spiritual search because it is deeply embedded in our psyche. One suggests the possibility that we are indeed 'wired for God'[6] with neuronal networks which enable us to specifically seek and find altered or transcendent states of consciousness, and which help us to find meaning and grounding in an often apparently meaningless and disorientating existence. Hamer[7] finds evidence of a genetic influence. An atheistic evolutionary cause is postulated in which spirituality and religiosity have survival advantages. The argument goes that being alive and aware of death can be so terrifying that belief, for example in an afterlife or a loving universal power, enabled human beings to cope with the world and survive it better than those who did not. Thus down the long millennia, 'God' got wired into our neurological pathways because we needed him/her/it there. Of course, this explanation does not rule out the possibility of divine or supernatural intervention, or the possibility that the 'wiring' could be ordained in order to connect with the absolute. In the first scenario, God or the Source of All is no more than a by-product of evolutionary processes, a mere figment of mental conjuring embedded in our genes to keep us safe. In the second the divine is very real and our whole make-up is geared to seeking that truth. Whichever perspective is accepted, human beings seem to have spirituality at the very core of their existence. It is part of what it is to be human, and as human beings we must inevitably, at some level, bring this into all aspects of our lives, including work. Indeed, in Western culture where adherence to the formal religions (q.v.) has nose-dived, our spiritual needs must be met in other milieu – such as personal relationships and work. Further, without religious adherence it may be argued that these may in future become our primary context for spiritual deepening.

Briskin[3] suggests that any kind of work which is devoid of meaning is ultimately dispiriting and destructive, and has partly been fuelled by the Industrial Revolution, when work, which had hitherto been largely rural and in small units or self-directed and agricultural, lost its relational quality. People no longer had control over their patterns of work but became caught up as cogs in a machine. Work increasingly lost its sense of place in the scheme of things becoming more disconnected from the wider creation, from a sense of the sacred. This phenomenon seems to have infiltrated all areas of working life. Whether commercial or public enterprises, small or large, charitable or profit making, there are variations in the symptoms but they are variations on a theme – the overall picture is one of dis-ease, disconnection and dissatisfaction at work rooted in an absence of spiritually nurturing relationships and connection to work at many levels.

Right relationship and the spiritually healthy workplace

I can remember the grainy black and white pictures of television in my post-war childhood, and *The Lone Ranger*, a popular western at the time, would see me glued before the screen. An old joke in business circles refers to the heroic Lone Ranger and his faithful Indian sidekick Tonto. Surrounded by hostile tribes, moving in for the kill, the Lone Ranger turns to Tonto and says, 'Well, looks like we've had it this time Tonto.' To which his faithful sidekick replies, 'What's this "we" business?'

Many people at work sometimes feel their relationships function like this. Relationships are not always as supportive as they might be. Many studies have illuminated how relationships at work are really power struggles rather than the collaborative efforts of supportive and egalitarian teams (see, for example, Hugman's[8] work among healthcare professionals). Disconnection can seep into every aspect of the workplace, dumbing down human relationships into perfunctory superficiality, battles of egos and the compulsion for instant gratification. The relationships at work mirror the nature of the corporate body. Disconnected organisations produce a disconnected workforce. Disconnected people produce disconnected organisations. And it could be argued that this in turn mirrors the disconnection some workers might feel within themselves – from their sense of centre, their highest or deepest self, the soul.

In such a culture, there is little room for the 'softer' things that seem to matter to people. Power struggles, an overweening attention to systems of control, top-down decision making, staff alienated from the decision-making process, emphasis on production and outcomes rather than process and relationality, lack of resources to do the job – these and other factors are well documented in the numerous studies on sickness, absenteeism, attrition rates and stress in the workplace. The impact on employees is higher levels of depression, hopelessness, despair, poor concentration and decision making, absenteeism, conflicts at home, physical illnesses, addiction to drugs and alcohol, and suicide, and on employers a significant escalation in their running costs.[9–17] The UK economy, for example, is believed to be losing in excess of £4 billion annually in such costs and one report suggests that each NHS trust is losing on average £450 000 a year in stress-related absence.[18] Meanwhile high-profile reports in the media have indicated successful prosecutions of organisations that fail to reduce stress on their staff – an employer has a duty of care to employees to prevent harm from stress.[16]

A couple of years ago I was involved in conducting a piece of research for the Royal College of Nursing (RCN),[19] which included a series of focus group exercises embracing over 2000 RCN members. A common thread was the sense of alienation from the workplace, which many nurses were, and still are, experiencing.

If spirituality means anything, it is about a sense of connection – with ourselves, each other, work and home, and that which is beyond the self – whatever we perceive it to be. Dispirited workplaces create a sense of separation and disconnection, we become divorced from the satisfaction of a job well done and of a sense of right relationship with those we seek to serve – be they patients, clients, customers – and our colleagues. Dispirited organisations are far more likely to have higher levels of sickness and absenteeism and, in the case of healthcare, more patient dissatisfaction and greater risks of patient abuse. A disconnected workforce who cannot find their heart and soul in their work are far more likely to shut down from the task, to defend themselves from the perceived anxiety of their work, to see the recipients of care as demanding from or attacking them. All of this conspires to produce settings that increase the likelihood of poor standards of care and even abuse.[20]

Many factors can contribute to this sense of disconnection, and one of them is the signal given to staff through the language that is dominant in the organisation. The RCN study showed how nurses particularly loathed much of the terminology that pervades modern healthcare. Since the time of the study, I have shared its findings with many groups of different health professionals, and it seems that nurses are not alone in this aversion. All kinds of therapists, doctors and other health and social service workers feel alienated by the language used to govern the work they do. 'Reports, meetings, conferences, it was suggested, speak of "key people" (but is not "every member of staff a key person?") or use the language of the business world ("take forward", "downsizing", "cost-effectiveness", "value for money", "evidence-based practice", "benchmarking", "business plans", "human resources") ... these and many others emerged as pet hates of respondents.'[19] The language we use in our services transmits all kinds of conscious and unconscious signals that influence the way people feel in the workplace. Language that sees people as resources, or caring work as targets, reduces the humanity of the context and contributes to the underlying sense of alienation that many feel at work. It is difficult to find our heart and soul being welcome in such a context. Work that should or could be enchanting, inspiring and sacred, where human beings can willingly give of their best, becomes disenchanting, dispiriting and desecrated. Work like this becomes deeply discouraging. The word 'discourage' has its roots in the French 'coeur' – heart. A workplace that nourishes and supports us is encouraging – literally has 'heart' in it.

There is compelling evidence, as suggested above, that the need for spiritual fulfilment is an integral part of being human. But is this something that should be left to the individual in their private time or is there a place for business, or any employing organisation for that matter, to take more of an interest or indeed action? Zohar and Marshall[21] say that individuals and organisations that possess 'spiritual intelligence', that is to say, actively seek, encourage and achieve meaning, purpose, connection, involvement and wholeness in all aspects of their being, are more likely to be happy, healthy and successful. Most employing organisations in commercially developed countries are bound by law to take care of their staff physically, mentally, socially and economically. But if spirituality is part of what it is to be human as well, just like our physiology and psychology, then it seems rational to presume that employers have a duty to support their staff in this dimension as well. Are we far off legislation compelling employers to meet certain spiritual needs of staff, just as in many places they are compelled to provide minimum wages or pensions? Is the day close when employers will be sued by unhappy employees who became depressed because of the aggravation of a sense of disconnectedness at work through not being involved in decisions about their working lives? Are we close to trade unions pressing employers to set up quiet sanctuaries in the workplace for meditation, prayer and reflection?

Goleman's thesis[22] showed that organisations with what he called 'emotional intelligence', that is, a sense of shared meaning, purpose, values and positive relationships at work, were far more likely to succeed. Likewise a Gallup report[23] found the most profitable and/or successful organisations were more likely to be those who actively promoted spiritual values and practices in the workplace. Thus a picture begins to emerge suggesting that enterprising and energetic companies and other organisations are likely to succeed in their goals when they pay attention to soul first and systems second. Such entities are likely to be even more successful when they adopt approaches that nourish the spirits as well as the salaries of their staff.

This means a lot more than investing in a crèche, better pay scales and access to aerobics or massage for the workers. Yet it doesn't have to cost a lot, and the methods available have been tried and tested throughout history: providing mentoring, support and spiritual counselling in the workplace; developing practices that support personal spiritual awareness, such as meditation; building communities and ways of conducting ourselves at work that generate a sense of support and connection. Add to these team-building exercises, time out together, access to rest and recuperation facilities, time for reflection and other techniques that deepen personal insights, motivation and the positive aspects of working relationships with colleagues and the organisation as a whole, and that which lies beyond the organisation. All of these and more[2,24] are directed towards encouraging a sense of meaning and purpose in the workplace and are focused on what right relationships, truth and highest values mean to people; how the goals of the organisation can be wedded to success without sacrificing kindness and compassion, welfare for other human beings and indeed all of creation. Matthew Fox[5] believes the task that lies ahead of us is enormous, because he calls for nothing less than a complete re-enchantment of the workplace and a re-consecration of work. A sceptic may balk at these words. Can the drudgery of work that so many know day in and day out ever be seen and felt as holy? It is easy to see this might be so for people like myself who have the privilege of doing work that is fulfilling. My work allows me considerable personal control, and I can weave my spiritual life into it so that any sense of being spiritual in some things and not in others simply disappears. How much more difficult must it be for the woman on the production line or the child in the sweatshop or the man down the pit? Work that offers a deep sense of spirituality – purpose, meaning, fulfilment, connected to 'all that is', serving God, however we experience it – currently seems to be an opportunity only for a minority because of the way much of our economy and social structures are organised. In this context, Matthew Fox's urgings are revolutionary and will demand nothing less than a complete rethink of the way we organise human activity. Meanwhile, an old saying holds true, 'nobody ever died wishing they had spent more time at the office'.

Most workers in Britain, and perhaps worldwide, would understand how Sisyphus felt. Condemned by the gods, his task was to eternally roll a huge boulder uphill. Labouring to the point of collapse, he would complete his struggle, only to see the boulder roll downhill again, and for him once more to repeat his labour. It doesn't have to be like this. We can be enterprising and efficient and still work from an ethical and spiritual basis in harmony with the workforce, society and the wider creation. There is hope for this, as many organisations that are choosing to work ethically and spiritually are demonstrating. Lerner[4] leaves us with an optimistic message suggesting that the old way of working will pass. History tells us that nothing lasts for long:

> It will pass because people hunger for a deeper kind of recognition from each other than the current organisation of society allows. It will change because people hunger for lives in which their spiritual needs are not just relegated to the sidelines and to their weekends, but rather fully expressed and integrated into our daily lives. It will change because people need to live in a world based on love and on caring for each other. It will change because people are coming to recognise the intrinsic connection between the ecological crisis and the values of individualism and selfishness enshrined in the competitive market. It will change because people need a world whose social institutions are based on a joint sense of awe and wonder at the universe and on a collective understanding of our role as stewards of and nurturers of Gaia. It will change because people will take their own understanding of the Unity of All Being seriously. (p.238)

Recent research indicates that the change is indeed under way, at least in Western culture.[25,26] For example, Heelas *et al.*[25] demonstrate the 'subjective turn' of the past 50 years or so in our culture, a characteristic of which had hitherto been a tendency for people to identify themselves according to objective, externally defined criteria – established ways of doing things, deference to authority, acceptance of certain truths (e.g. the superiority of men, professionals and so on) – as givens. The steady death of our way of defining our place in the world in this way is characterised in the 'subjective turn' – a cultural shift where we seek inner understanding, exploration of self, personal experience of the world and so on.

This has led to changes in organisational emphases – including those concerned with caring work. It was always doctor, nurse, social worker, teacher, etc., knows best. Now it is patient- or client-centred care, charters, rights, partnership and involvement. Health and social care workers have been caught up in this shift into what Heelas *et al.* call the 'holistic milieu', for they have taken the subjective turn too. Surrender to authority is no longer acceptable if holistic, person-centred care is to be possible. Yet many carers find themselves trapped in organisations that do not foster the holistic milieu, such as the NHS. And while they may lay claim to caring for staff and patients, in reality our health institutions incline towards the 'iron cage of bureaucracy' model, and targets dominate life. Heelas *et al.* go on to suggest that after some time trying to accommodate the iron cage, many staff give up and go part time, or leave to find some environment more in tune with their subjective needs. Heart and soul at work is an integral part of the holistic milieu. At the moment there seems to be a kind of spiritual jet lag at work in many of our health and social care organisations – they have not yet caught up with the aspirations of their workforces rooted in the massive subjective turn which the past 50 years or so have witnessed.

The re-enchantment of work

Making work a place with heart and soul does not have to be complicated, nor does it have to be expensive. For example, some units used for development work in the NHS often had higher workloads, yet sickness, absenteeism and attrition rates were less.[27,28] Why? Because the staff working in them were more supportive of each other, had a shared sense of mission and purpose in their work, and a deeper sense of connection with each other, which made the work culture more soulful, more satisfying. Dispirited workforces, as I have explored above, are a disaster for the individuals who work in them, for the teams and for those who depend on them for care.

From the research I have cited in this chapter (summarised[2,29]), many options for making work more soulful are well identified and have been used with success in many settings (Box 6.1).

Box 6.1   Options for making work more soulful

- Setting up shared educational programmes
- Proper resources for staff to do the job, and systems in place to check this
- Reflective practice, clinical supervision, mentoring
- Social events
- Multidisciplinary projects
- Pre- and post-shift debriefings
- Team-building sessions
- Shared exploration of boundaries and working practices
- Developing and implementing anti-bullying policies
- Networking and learning sets with groups with similar interests
- Using email networks, staff journals, etc., to ensure everyone knows what's going on
- Staff involvement in decision making at every level
- Stress management education
- Introducing relaxation techniques for staff such as meditation training, tai chi, complementary therapies, etc.
- Creating quiet 'sanctuaries' where staff can be in silence away from work
- Access to independent/spiritual counselling
- Leadership development

These are just a few examples of the many possibilities available, which have been used with some success in a wide range of settings, according to the reports. What seems to work best is a comprehensive strategy, not just providing employee-friendly policies *or* staff counselling *or* team-building days *or* better personal exercise – but embracing all of these and more. The more comprehensive the strategy, the more it is likely to be successful in building a sense of connection and right relationship in the workplace and making work a great place to be, as well as do. The cultivation of right relationships between the organisation and those it employs, among teams and the individual employee's sense of being in right relationship with the self, are key levels of concern. The interplay of the relationships between the individual's inner experience – how I feel about myself, how grounded and 'at one' with the world I am – and the quality of relationships in teams and the wider organisation are the seedbed for soul-full workplaces.

Individuals, teams and organisations each have a part to play. At the same time it is important to be gentle on ourselves and remember that we don't have to have everything perfectly in place. Creating a soulful community is forever 'work in progress', for there will always be challenges, errors and the shadows in our unconscious to be resolved. An incremental approach would seem to be the most appropriate – the more bits of the jigsaw puzzle are in place, the more complete the picture, but it does not have to be done all at once. For example, it may not be possible to do much about the wider workplace culture, but could something be done to enhance support in the team, such as implementing reflective practice? Could an individual do something like take up meditation? Starting small by tackling one or two achievable issues first that can make a difference, is a more realistic and healthy approach.

In summary, the main points can be grouped under four main themes if the workplace is to be ensouled.

1 Soul friends: access to the support of one or more wise counsellors or mentors to provide ongoing guidance, mentoring and spiritual counselling to individuals, teams and organisations – these are skilled people who have walked the path before and are themselves rich in understanding and experience of spirituality.
2 Soul communities: safe groups of people who nourish ongoing spiritual awakening. It might be a fellow group of meditators, a reflective practice group at work, a church group and so on, there are many possibilities. With time and commitment the workplace itself can emerge as a soul community.
3 Soul foods: through the inspiration of poetry, music, art, nature, scripture and so on that refresh, renew and revitalise.
4 Soul works: developing spiritual practices which nurture and develop the individual and collective spirit – meditation, prayer, yoga, the Enneagram (a personality inventory which incorporates spiritual guidance[30]), retreat time, tai chi and so on, the list is endless. Practical things that can be done, some alone, some in groups with the soul community.

Spirituality needs to be practised. It is not just a private indulgence, but goes further and is acted out in the world. Each working moment can also be an opportunity for 'soul growth', just like growth in our relationships. We may undertake specific spiritual practices (worship through prayer or practise meditation, for example), but our everyday work is pregnant with spiritual potential too. It provides us with countless teachings each day, about others and ourselves. It confronts us with endless challenges to care in settings and relationships that may be hostile to caring. It opens windows for us into the absolute, whatever that means for us, where we seek and find answers to the meaning of our lives, often in moments of great challenge and suffering.

All the great spiritual traditions speak of the path of service. Pursuing the inner work to discover right relationship with ourselves, and perhaps our God, may become a kind of spiritual self-gratification if it does not manifest itself in the world in some way. Whether we adopt a theistic or atheistic world-view, the message is the same – to deepen our understanding of ourselves and our part in the scheme of things, but at some point integrate this and apply it in our life and work. Thus, the occupation of the carer can provide an ideal opportunity to bring more love and compassion into the world through the relief of suffering. And it is compassion without attachment – a way of being in the world that does not exhaust us with the burden of caring for others, but which liberates us to care from a place of resting at home within ourselves.

Valuing our own work of caring and recognising its essentially sacred nature is perhaps the most important thing we can do towards restoring the sacred to caring. What we do is significant, it matters, and coming to accept that, when we so often undervalue the contribution we make, is part of the process of getting into right relationship. Our work provides us with the milieu for action in the world. Valuing it, being in right relationship with it, helps us toward right relationship with ourselves. Anyone in caring work is blessed, in that sense, by not having to go out and find work of compassionate service. We are in it already, all we have to do is approach it more consciously. The collective enterprise of ensouling the workplace is a true gift to humanity in health and social services. It is the milieu in which suffering is alleviated through the individual and group experience of work that is open to heart and soul.

In a culture that has rendered so much of work to the completion of limited functions or perfunctory performance targets, the pursuit of spirituality can seem a hopeless delusion in the face of the enormity of the shift that is required. Yet as we have seen from the many studies and examples cited above, there are strong signs that this shift is under way. In that there lies hope, and hope is the food of the soul. As Matthew Fox[5] observes:

> Is this not the source of all good work – to make manifest our being and our loving in our livelihood? And the joy that we are promised by starting work all over again will itself give us the energy to carry on the task. The universe is asking a great task of us today; it is extending to us a pressing invitation to reconnect out daily lives to the Great Work of the universe. New vocations, new callings, new roles are everywhere in the air. New work awaits. The harvest is greater than the number of labourers. Are we listening? Are we willing? Can we say to the beloved, 'I am here, I am willing'? (p.307)

References

1 Aquinas T, cited in Fox M (1992) *Sheer Joy: conversations with Thomas Aquinas on creation spirituality*. Harper, San Francisco, CA, p.256.
2 Wright SG, Sayre-Adams J (2001) *Sacred Space – right relationship and spirituality in healthcare*. Churchill Livingstone, London.
3 Briskin A (1998) *The Stirring of Soul in the Workplace*. Berrett-Koehler, San Francisco, CA.
4 Lerner M (2000) *Spirit Matters*. Hampton Roads, Charlottesville, Virginia.
5 Fox M (1994) *The Reinvention of Work – a new vision of livelihood for our time*. Harper, San Francisco, CA.
6 Newberg A, D'Aquili E, Rause V (2001) *Why God Won't Go Away*. Ballantine, New York, NY.

7   Hamer D (2004) *The God Gene*. Doubleday, New York, NY.

8   Hugman R (1991) *Power in Caring Professions*. Macmillan, London.

9   Borrill C, Wall T, West M *et al.* (1998) *Mental Health of the Workforce in NHS Trusts*. Institute of Work Psychology, University of Sheffield.

10   Williams S, Mitchie S, Pattani S (1998) *Improving the Health of the NHS Workforce*. Nuffield, London.

11   World Health Organization (1994) *Guidelines for the Primary Prevention of Mental, Neurological and Psychosocial Disorders (5) – Staff Burnout*. WHO Division of Mental Health No. who/mnh/mnd/94.21, Geneva.

12   Health Education Authority (1996) *Organisational Stress*. HEA, London.

13   Health Education Authority (1998) *More Than Brown Bread and Aerobics*. HEA, London.

14   Health and Safety Executive (2004) Data taken from website January 2004. www.hse.gov.uk/statistics/pdf/swi04.pdf.

15   Confederation of British Industry (CBI) (1999) *Promoting Mental Health at Work*. CBI, London.

16   Health and Safety Executive (2005) Data taken from website April 2005. www.hse.gov.uk/stress.

17   Snow C, Willard P (1989) *I'm Dying to Take Care of You*. Professional Counsellor Books, Redmond, New Jersey.

18   Gooding L (2005) Stress poses dire threat to NHS. *Nursing Standard*. **19**(21): 4.

19   Wright S, Gough P, Poulton B (1998) *Imagining the Future* (full report). RCN, London.

20   Obholzer A, Roberts V (eds) (2003) *The Unconscious at Work*. Brunner-Routledge, New York, NY.

21   Zohar D, Marshall I (2000) *Spiritual Intelligence the Ultimate Intelligence*. Bloomsbury, London.

22   Goleman D (1995) *Emotional Intelligence*. Bantam, New York, NY.

23   Gallup Organisation, survey cited in Hatfield D (1999) New research links emotional intelligence with profitability. *The Inner Edge*. **1**(5): 5–9.

24   Wright SG (2005) *Reflections on Spirituality and Health*. Whurr, London.

25   Heelas P, Woodhead L, Seel B *et al.* (2005) *The Spirituality Revolution – why religion is giving way to spirituality*. Blackwell, Oxford.

26   Tacey D (2000) *The Spiritual Revolution*. Harpercollins, Sydney.

27   Salvage J, Wright SG (1996) *Nursing Development Units – a force for change*. Scutari, London.

28   Page S (ed.) (1998) *Practice Development Units*. Arnold, London.

29   Wright SG (2005) *Burnout – a spiritual crisis*. RCN/Nursing Standard Supplements, London.

30   Riso D, Hudson R (1999) *The Wisdom of the Enneagram*. Bantam, New York, NY.

Religious, philosophical and cultural considerations

CHAPTER 7

Faith and experience: paradigms of spirituality

Burkhard Scherer

Introduction

This chapter provides an overview and interpretation of forms of spirituality as found in different religious traditions, and their relevance in care. It therefore aims to raise awareness of different forms of spirituality, attempts to convey a sense of similarities and differences between these, and highlights the impact of different forms of spirituality on care. It comprises four parts.

- Religion and spirituality – these are addressed theoretically. The history and philosophy behind the term 'religion' is explored. Different theories and definitions of 'religion' are considered. The term 'spirituality' is then integrated into this theoretical discussion.
- Classification of religions – different classifications of religions and spiritualities will be explained and a phenomenological approach utilising the polar paradigms of 'faith' and 'experience' emerges.
- Are religions good? Inter-religious dialogue is discussed in relation to tolerance in democratic culture.
- Spiritualities in context – different spiritual attitudes are exemplified and analysed in context; the implications of the findings for care are considered.

Religion and spirituality

When talking about 'spirituality' and 'religion', it is important to be conscious about the implications for interpretation (hermeneutic implications) and limits of the usage of these terms. 'Spirituality' is a sensitive term in that it can be interpreted in both a broader and more specific way than the term 'religion'. On the one hand, 'spirituality' points to what could be described as entailing certain dimensions of religion, especially the ritual and the experiential dimensions in the typologies of Smart, which will be introduced in more detail later[1,2] (Smart, pp.11–22). On the other hand, spirituality can also comprise religious expressions outside the boundaries of institutionalised religion (alternative religiosity),[3] and even human expressions outside any explicitly religious context (secular religion).[4,5] It can then be seen as human questions around uncertainty and the meaning of existence. Spirituality is also found in the ritualisations and mythologies of popular culture, especially

Internet, film and television (popular religion).[6] This is similarly exemplified in *'Star Trek* religion', with its Klingon weddings, dress conventions and the occasional cult of the Bajoran prophets.[7,8] Before we attempt to understand religion-based spirituality, we need to investigate what 'religion' implies, both historically and philosophically.

Antiquity

In Greco-Roman antiquity[9,10] (Figl, pp.63–4), the Latin term *'religio'* referred mainly to the social and ritual dimensions of religion. The verb *'re-ligere'*, from which the noun *'religio'* is derived, means indeed 'to conscientiously fulfil one's own duty in the (state) cult'. The adjective *religiosus*, on the other hand, reflects a preoccupation with cultic matters and assumes the meaning 'superstitious'. The contrast between religious duty and superstition is expressed by Nigidius Figulus (*ca.* 100–45BC or Before Common Era/BCE), who, together with Varro and Cicero, figures among the greatest savants of his time:

> One must fulfil one's own duty in the cult conscientiously in order not to become scared and superstitious (*religiosus*).[11]

Also in the first century BCE, Cicero proposed a Roman philosophical etymology of the term *'religio'*. Deriving it from the verb *'relegere'* (to read again and again), he interpreted it as 'carefully ponder the sacred matters'.[12] This interpretation relates mainly to the philosophical dimension of religion. Later, in Christian antiquity, *religio* came to be understood as the expression of the relationship between humans and the divine (in Christianity: God). In 305AD (or Common Era/CE), Lactantius derived the term *'religio'* from the verb *'religari'*, meaning 'to reconnect oneself; to be reconnected to (God)'.[13] Interestingly, the prefix *'re-'* shifts here in its meaning from 'again and again' to 'carefully' towards 'once again', already presupposing a primordial state of wholeness (in Christian terms: paradise before the fall of men); hence, 'religion' reconnects sinning mankind with the lost paradise. Leaving the Christian subtext aside, the understanding of 'religion' as 'ligion', that is, as link between the human and the metaphysical ('beyond natural' or 'beyond human/supernatural') world still remains – despite its limitations – one of the most commonly employed working definitions of 'religion'.

From the Middle Ages to German Idealism

In the Christian Middle Ages the meaning of *religio* had shifted again. *Religio* now denoted the monastic class, with *religiosus* being a member of that class. The terms faith (*fides*), law (*lex*) or confession (*secta*) were used in contexts where the term 'religion' in its modern meaning applies. Finally, after the reformation (sixteenth century CE), *religio* came to denote a system of doctrines, and by the Age of Enlightenment (seventeenth century CE) the term 'natural Religion' was coined by Herbert of Cherbury[9,10,14] to denote the following:

- existence of God
- worship of God

- virtue and piety
- remorse and penance for sins
- reward and punishment in the afterlife.

In the philosophy of German Idealism (eighteenth/nineteenth century, roughly from Kant to Schopenhauer), the nature of the divine or God became more the focus of philosophical critique. Immanuel Kant (1724–1804) contributed greatly to the understanding of religion by making God a demand of practical reason, and thereby reduced 'religion' to its ethical dimension. As warrant of morality, God is not susceptible to empirical proof. This leads ultimately to positivism – the view that whatever you claim to be true (the existence of a soul, of God, etc.) needs to be rationally and scientifically provable or verifiable. This view was promoted by philosophers such as Francis Bacon, David Hume and above all August Comte (1798–1857), the father of modern sociology. In the sociology of religion as established by Durkheim (1858–1917), the focus of investigation was not concerned with its alleged connection to the supernatural but solely the function of religion as a social entity. On the other hand, the romanticist theologian Schleiermacher (1768–1834) considered religion an 'expression of the feeling of absolute dependence' towards God. His thoughts remain most influential in the work of modern theologians such as Barth and Tillich.

Nineteenth to twentieth century

One of many modern disciplines of humanities, religious studies became properly established in the nineteenth century. Approaches to religious theory varied and constituted one of the following.

- Developmental or evolutionist – viewed religion as a phenomenon in human history.
- Functionalist – considered the function of religion for the individual or society.
- Substantialistic – alleged 'essence' of religion[10] (pp.65–8).

Evolutionist thinkers include the father of cultural anthropology, Tylor (1832–1917), who considered a belief in spirits, known as animism, to be the original form of religion; and the anthropologist and classical scholar Frazer (1854–1941), who believed magic was the primitive form and predecessor of religion.

Functionalistic theories consider religion either from a sociological (Durkheim, see above) or psychological perspective. For instance, Freud (1856–1939) explains religion as expression of infantile dependence and wishful thinking. Jung's (1875–1961) view is that religion is an elaborate expression of what he called the 'collective unconscious': an unconscious substratum of experience and thoughts common to all human beings. Functionalistic theories still in use include psychological and socio-biological approaches.[15]

Substantialistic theories maintain that all religions have a common essence; for instance, they share a belief in supernatural forces (e.g. Tylor's spiritual beings), in 'power' (Söderblom, 1866–1931) or as experience of superior power (van der Leeuw, 1850–1950). One of the most influential of these theorists, Rudolf Otto (1869–1937), believing the essence of religions to be the irrational dimension in human life, introduced the term 'sacred' to describe the abstract substance of religion. The 'sacred' dominated religious studies in the twentieth century, especially through the work of Mircea Eliade.[16] Mensching (1901–1978)[17] also defines 'religion' using the term sacred:

> Religion is encounter with the Sacred through experience and the responsive acting of the human who is determined by the Sacred. (p.15)

Modern approaches

In modern religious studies there are many definitions of religion. Already at the beginning of the twentieth century, Leuba[10] (p.62) grouped definitions into three approaches – intellectualistic, emotional and voluntaristic (related to the will and power of mind). A good example of a useful modern approach is Geertz's[18] (p.4) culturalistic synthesis, which defines religion as:

- a system of symbols which acts to:
  - establish powerful, pervasive and long-lasting moods and motivations in men by
  - formulating conceptions of a general order of existence and
  - clothing these conceptions with such an aura of factuality that
  - the moods and motivations seem uniquely realistic.

Despite an abundance of working models, postmodernism and deconstructivism deny religion as a definable concept. WC Smith[19] (pp.50, 156, 195) demonstrated the term 'religion' to be confusing, superfluous, and distorting, believing 'religion' to be better described as 'cumulative tradition' and 'faith'. And JZ Smith[20] (p.xi) maintains:

> There is no data for religion. Religion is solely the creation of the scholar's study.

Society has become increasingly sensitive to the problem of Western colonialism and the romantic misunderstanding of Eastern cultures. This is also relevant to the utilisation of the term 'religion' itself.[21] Also, religion is depicted as an intellectual invention of modernity[22] (p.23), and the postmodern deconstruction of the term 'religion' results in, terminologically, irresolvable doubt (*aporia*).

However, the pluralism of perspectives, which comes out of postmodern thought, is a welcome enrichment when exploring religions and spirituality[10] (pp.72–3). This is best served by a multidimensional understanding of religions.

The many dimensions of religions

Modern study of religion reflects a consensus in approaching this human phenomenon multidimensionally and is exemplified in the seven dimensions of religions developed by Smart (1928–2001).[1] His categories provide a tool for the empirical analysis of religions rather than pretending to define religions in their totalities or to reduce them to a single common denominator (Box 7.1).

Box 7.1   Seven dimensions of religions[2]

1 ritual/practical
2 doctrinal/philosophical
3 mythic/narrative
4 experiential/emotional
5 ethical/legal
6 organisational/social
7 material/artistic

In applying Smart's dimensions to the analysis of different religions, for example Christianity and Buddhism[23] (pp.364–73), the differences and commonalities of philosophy and practice become evident.

The ritual dimension expresses itself in Christianity in, for example, liturgy and sacramental rites such as baptism. In contrast Buddhism has less institutionalised rituality, although rites are performed, for example, at the ordination of a monk.

The doctrinal dimension in Christianity is expressed in its dogmas, or teachings, such as the incarnation or the trinity. These teachings are the result of a philosophical-theological process in the first centuries of the existence of Christianity. In Buddhism, the teachings of the Buddha form the philosophical foundations for engaging in a gradual experiential transformation of awareness into enlightenment. Hence philosophy, not dogma, lies at the core of Buddhism.

The Biblical narratives constitute the mythic dimension in Christianity. The accounts about Jesus of Nazareth form the foundation of the Christian faith, whereby Jesus's life is interpreted as central for the salvation of humankind. Myths seem to play a less dominant role in the canons of Buddhism and where they occur, they are generally only considered as meaningful as far as they encourage people to make their own experiences.

Despite a long history of contemplation in Christian monasticism, mainstream Christianity discouraged immediate experience of the divine in the form of mysticism and encouraged mere devotion within an unsurpassable hierarchical structure (God – Church – individual). Buddhism, on the contrary, is all about experiencing for oneself. Without personal experience in the form of meditation, there is no spiritual development in Buddhism. The goal of Buddha's path is enlightenment – the experience of things how they really are.

The ethical dimension of Christianity is laid down by the new interpretation of the Jewish Law (Torah) – especially the Ten Commandments – by Jesus of Nazareth, Paul of Tharsos (St Paul) and others. Buddhism entails extensive rules for nuns and monks and elaborate ethical guidelines for laypersons, which emphasise self-responsibility and insight rather than sinfulness and punishment.

Organisationally, Christianity tends to be centrally and hierarchically structured, as can be seen in the Roman Catholic Church; disagreements in doctrines and practice led to exclusive and often hostile denominations. Buddhism has diversified peacefully, developing a variety of approaches towards the Buddha's teachings, each valuable in itself and mutually accepting. Schools and congregations have developed independent structures.

Artistically, Christianity and Buddhism are expressed in monumental works of arts, architecture, literature and music, each reflecting or challenging the other religious dimensions (especially the ritual, doctrinal, narrative and experiential dimensions).

Spirituality

Although we might carry an unresolved doubt about what a 'religion' actually is, with Smart's toolbox we are enabled to portray religious phenomena quite sufficiently. By analogy, 'spirituality' can be approached by using the same categories with maybe a shift of emphasis from institutionalised to personalised religious expression. It seems that 'spirituality', although possibly informed by an institutional and legal dimension, centres on personal and individual responses towards questions of existence and meaning. The term broadens to include alternative religiosity such as New Age, Esotericism and Hermetism, most of which are roughly characterised by a healthy mistrust of religious authorities. Further, spirituality also pertains to secular responses to existential questions and even human expressions outside any explicitly religious context, which nonetheless can be meaningfully interpreted using terms such as 'secular' or 'implicit' religion.[24] Secular spirituality is found in 'hidden religions' (crypto-religions), systems which pretend not to be religious while displaying characteristics of religions, such as the dominant extreme ideologies of the twentieth century, fascism and communism. It is also found in the rituals and mythologies of popular culture, especially Internet, film and television, which provide 'popular religion' as a spiritual home for the masses. This applies not only to modern mythologies such as the aforementioned *Star Trek* or *Lord of the Rings*, but also to the rituals and symbols among sports supporters, which constitute systems of symbols functioning according to Geertz's culturalistic definition of religion (see above).

With this in mind, let us proceed to chart religions according to the most standardised spiritual responses they provoke: faith and experience.

Classification of religion

There is no universally accepted classification within the academic study of religions. Major religions are variously grouped together, for instance geographically as Western versus Eastern traditions, for example by Oxtoby[25] (pp.4–5). Here, 'Western traditions' relates mainly to Judaism, Christianity and Islam, while 'Eastern traditions' denotes religions originating in India and China, such as Hinduism, Buddhism and Daoism. This classification has the advantage that it avoids implicit judgements on the nature of the religions in question; however, the geographical angle is somewhat arbitrary and limiting. Traditions like Sikhism, which originate in India, but owe a great deal to the 'Western' tradition of Islam, are not readily described by either term; nor does the juxtaposition 'Eastern'–'Western' give real justice to the peculiarities of, for example, Christianity and Islam in their Asian adaptations or the neo-religious movements originating in South and East Asia spreading into the West. This classification becomes even more problematic when talking about ancient world religions with strong histories in both Europe and Asia, such as Manichaeism. The list of problem cases could be easily extended.

Even more narrowing is the application of historical terms such as 'Abrahamic' versus 'Asian' or 'Indian traditions'. The latter terms are broad enough to entail any religious tradition in, or originating from, Asia or India, which consequently need to include traditions such as Sikhism or Indian Islam and Asian Christianity, all of which can be classified as 'Abrahamic'.

The term 'Abrahamic' denotes the three major religions, which originated in the ancient Near East: Judaism, Christianity and Islam. Their adherents comprise roughly half of the world population. The Abrahamic religions share the patriarch Abraham as their ancestor and they are commonly characterised by the belief in one God, or monotheism, and in the case of Christianity in the paradoxical formula of one God in three persons. Since these religions are not the only monotheistic traditions in the world, for example there are monotheistic Hindu traditions, they are quite rightly called desert monotheist traditions (pointing to their origin in the Arabic desert). Another good alternative term is 'elective monotheism', since this term combines the notion of one creator God with the notion of a 'chosen people' that is so important to Judaism and subsequently redefined by Christianity and Islam.[26]

'Abrahamic' is problematic for many reasons. First of all, the role of Abraham in the design of each religion is quite differently weighed. In Christianity, Abraham plays a significantly smaller role than in Judaism and Islam. Still, Christian theologians, such as Küng and Kuschel, use the term to construct an 'Abrahamic ecumene' – a level of unity of Judaism, Christianity and Islam.[27] The sense of community of these three traditions is well meant, but is nevertheless quite flawed. For instance, Muslims object to the term 'Abrahamic religion' being applied to Judaism and Christianity, since in their conviction Islam is the only true Abrahamic religion,[28] and Judaism and Christianity, as 'religions of the book' (i.e. the Bible), possess only a degenerated version of the alleged one truth. Also, a variety of minor traditions such as Mandaeism, Sikhism, Druze, Bahá'í and Rastafarianism could be called Abrahamic in accordance with the doctrinal claims they make.

Instead of grouping religions historically or geographically, it is meaningful to describe religions according to their predominant characteristics, and therefore classify them phenomenologically. Comparative classifications have been introduced. The most prominent, by the sociologist Max Weber, constructed the conflicting ideal types of 'prophetic' and 'mystic' religion.

Prophetic religions, which include the desert monotheist religions but also others, such as Manichaeism and Zoroastrianism (Parsism), can be characterised by their claim of an absolute, revealed truth. A 'prophet' appears claiming to be in possession of an ultimate revelation. All questions about the meaning of life answered, adherents of prophetic religions are asked to believe in the revelation and act accordingly. Seeking, doubting, and trial and error are not part of their spirituality. The desert monotheist religions function as socio-religious contracts between the supernatural – an almighty creator god – and mankind or its elected part (for example, in Judaism). Humans follow God's revealed will and, quid pro quo, God protects them and rewards them in the afterlife. Consequently, in prophetic religions, we find the predominance of doctrine or faith, teleological, historical and tradition-oriented thinking, centrifugal activity (actions aim for an outer reality) and unfortunately the inclination to religious intolerance, holy wars, mission and proselytising.

On the other hand, 'mystic' religions propagate a spiritual path rather then a revealed ultimate truth. The revelation of ultimate reality is not clear-cut, but asserted as the goal of a spiritual path. Personal experience and spiritual development and transformation are more important than doctrines. Examples of these religions include most forms of Hinduism, Buddhism and Daoism, but also many 'primal religions' with mystic elements such as shamanism. They are characterised by the superiority of experience, non-historical and holistic world-views, centripetal activity (actions aim for an inner reality and transformation), and an inclusive, tolerant and non-proselytising view on other religions.

In faith religions, believers will never become what they believe in. For example, the soul will never be God. In experience religions, individuals will ultimately be transformed and become their goal, for example brahman or Buddha. Therefore faith religions have to be called dualistic – maintaining an ultimate duality of subject and object, creator and creation. Pure experience religions such as Buddhism and Advaita-('non-dual') Vedanta Hinduism are beyond this dualism. Perceiver, perceived and perception are one (Table 7.1).

Table 7.1 Comparing religions of faith and experience

Faith (in prophetic religions)	Experience (in mystic religions)
Doctrine, contract (covenant)	Path
Prayer	Meditation
Prophecy	Mystic
Outer revelation	Inner enlightenment
Linear historical thinking	Non-historical and holistic world-views
Centrifugal activity	Centripetal activity
Proselytising	Inner transformation
Excluding 'other truths', electiveness	Inclusive, tolerant
Dualistic (god – soul)	Non-dualistic

This phenomenological classification of religions into religions of faith versus religions of experience is valid in a very broad sense[29] (pp.16–18), [30] (pp.47–8). However, this classification may disregard aspects of either faith or mystic religion being present in a particular historical, social or personal aspect of labelled religions. For instance, there are strong cases to be made for spiritual experience in the form of mysticism within faith religions; but in Judaism, Christianity and Islam, mysticism never became mainstream religious expression. Mainstream Christianity and Islam, in particular, have treated mystics with open suspicion and often excommunicated, persecuted, killed or at least silenced mystics. Moreover, mystical experience within faith religions remains constrained by its doctrinal framework. The Christian *contemplatio* does not aim for total unity of the soul and its creator, Muslim *dhikr* remembers God's presence, but does not lead to total absorption into God. Structurally, faith religions favour dialogue with the absolute in prayer rather than immediate experience of the absolute in meditation.

On the other hand, faith can play a substantial role within experience religions, especially in folk religiosity. Trust and devotion (*shraddha* and *bhakti*) are conditions and methods of experience often required and employed in Indian and East Asian religions in order to engage on the path towards spiritual transformation, be that realising enlightenment, which is the full development of mind's potential, Buddhahood in Buddhism, or the liberating reintegration of the self (*atman*) into the Absolute (*brahman*) in mainstream Vedanta Hinduism.

Are religions good?

It is useful to dwell more on the understanding of truth in religion. This will prove important when we try and predict chances and limits of inter-religious dialogue, as well as those of personal expressions of spirituality.

Traditionally, most ancient religions defined themselves by utilising a dichotomy of pure versus impure in cult. In contrast, in desert monotheist traditions, we find the opposition 'true' and 'false' religion. This has been called the 'Mosaic distinction'.[31,32] The introduction of a binary category 'true' and 'false' has grave consequences, which can be described as the 'cost of monotheism': a proneness to religious intolerance and violence.[33,34]

A well-cherished, romantic assumption still prevailing in the current Inter-Faith and Global Ethics movement is the presupposition that all religions are good *per se*, and that hatred and violence conducted in the name of religions constitute perversions of religion. But, in fact, religions are neither good nor bad, they just 'are'. They can express themselves in both ways. In the same way, humans are neither good nor bad, neither difficult nor pleasant in an exclusive way. Still some religions are more prone to express themselves in an intolerant and violent way. This certainly depends on their understanding of (absolute) truth. He who possesses the 'only way', the 'truth' and the exclusive revelation is prone to persecute those who do not want to believe.

In inter-faith dialogue, 'truth' cannot play a meaningful role, since the acknowledgement of any ultimate truth presupposes a Kierkegaardian 'leap of faith' ('I believe therefore it is true'). Instead, in inter-religious dialogue, the main motivation should be ethical: how to achieve happiness for all within and even in spite of religions. Religions should ask themselves, whether they want to serve mankind or whether they expect mankind to serve them[35] (p.7). Accordingly, the free world should not tolerate religious expressions which suppress human rights in the name of any truth. In the face of current religious intolerance and fundamentalism, mainly from the desert monotheist side, pluralistic societies need to make the tough decision, whose choices they want to protect. This concerns the necessity of a 'fortified democracy', a concept developed by Jaspers[36] and famously summarised in the quotation: 'Democracy is tolerant towards all choices, but it must be able to become intolerant towards intolerance itself.'

Spiritualities in context

When classifying religions into either those of faith (such as Christianity and Islam) or experience (such as Buddhism), we have to keep in mind that individual spirituality may be expressed quite differently from mainstream institutionalised religiosity. When dealing with spirituality, for example, in the context of support work and healthcare, it is very important to treat clients as individuals with specific spiritual frames of mind that determine needs, rather than pigeon-holing them as a mere member of a religious tradition. On the other hand, recognising an individual's religious affiliation can provide a general frame within which individual spiritual expression can be expected to flourish. Therefore religious affiliation might be used as an initial indication of spiritual frame of mind, but not interpreted with rigid prescription.

It is helpful to contextualise spiritual needs across the religions. In faith religions, spirituality can centre on showing loyalty, for example towards the creator God. For instance, Muslims believe in God, His angels, His scriptures and His Messenger Muhammad, as well as in the day of judgement.[37] Muslims express their faith and submission to God's will (Islam means 'submission') through the ritual of prayer. This is appropriately called *salah*, meaning 'connection': it connects the believers with their object of faith. Muslims are supposed to conduct the *salah* five times a day. As a crucial expression of institutionalised Muslim spirituality, omitting these prayers can cause considerate distress to the faithful, although Muslim theology provides licences in case of travel and sickness. On the other hand, a semi-secular Muslim might prefer the personal prayer or *du'a* (meaning call) to the formal prayer duty. This often includes traditional or improvised praises (*tasbih*), spontaneously formulated or meditatively spoken with the aid of prayer beads.

In the face of sickness or death, a common spiritual response of Muslims is fatalism, submission to God's will; the Arabic expression *Insh-allah*, 'So God wills', characterises this attitude very well. Life is generally seen as a learning process and a trial, in which God sets tasks, blesses good actions, reprimands evil or, in the case of repentance, forgives. Here, supportive care can be constructive by drawing on the Islamic concept of God's mercifulness (*rahma*), and also by encouraging self-realisation: 'He who knows himself, knows God.[38]

In contrast, Buddhism, as a religion of experience, takes a radically different approach. It is not loyalty towards revealed doctrines but personal transformation that is the key role in this religion. Also, a Buddhist is one who meditates, not one who thinks 'Buddha is right'[39] (p.58). Of course, Buddhists trust in the Buddha as the teacher, who holds the mirror in which the mind's full development appears. This is a useful concept, but the Buddhist can doubt, and there is no limit to checking teachings against their own experience and common sense all the way till enlightenment. The Buddha called upon his followers not to 'come and believe' but to 'come and see for yourself' (*ehi passa*). Buddha's teachings are guidelines, some of which individual Buddhists will find personally useful, and others not. Having chosen, they work these guidelines within their own interests and capacities on the way to enlightenment. Very radically, in Buddhism, the truth of the Buddhist path is ultimately relative. It is like a raft over the river of conditioned reality: once the river is crossed, the raft is no longer needed[40,41] (pp.44–5). The real paradox then is that even where ultimate truth claims seem to be made in Buddhist schools, they are relative! And at the same time there is no place for a judging God or predestination and fate in Buddhism. There is just cause and effect (*karma*), a strictly logical natural law of 'what goes around comes around'. Former thoughts, words and actions became our present state. But this means that Buddhism takes our freedom of will seriously. No forgiving or punishing god can take away the consequences of our actions. At the same time, we are sowing now the seeds for our future. In the face of sickness and death, Buddhists can draw on their meditational practices and experiences. Physical obstacles are first-hand reminders of impermanence and a strong encouragement to use the precious opportunities to meditate while they last. Here, supportive care can be constructive by providing a quiet and peaceful atmosphere and facilitating or encouraging meditation. This is exemplified in the care of a dying Tibetan Buddhist (*see* Appendix).

Conclusion

Although the classification of religions presented remains a mere overview, 'faith' and 'experience' have been demonstrated to constitute meaningful paradigms for charting spiritual and religious views and expressions. Both polar categories provide us with a useful guide when approaching individual understandings and views on spirituality and religion. They also demonstrate points of potential conflict and tension between different religious convictions. Religious tolerance is a global, societal and individual issue. Additionally, it provides a starting point for some critical self-questioning, particularly relevant to the pressing global issue of religious tolerance: do we follow a suppressive or an empowering system? Can we excuse or condemn oppression and violence in the name of religions without excusing or condemning the typological matrix behind it?

In health and social care, a greater awareness of the historical roots and development of religions of faith and experience will help professionals understand the differing needs of those in their care in relation to professed religion but not negate the requirement for them to assess an individual's interpretation of religious practice.

References

1 Smart N (1996) *Dimensions of the Sacred. An Anatomy of World's Beliefs.* University of California Press, Berkeley, CA.
2 Smart N (1998) *The World's Religions* (2e). Cambridge University Press, Cambridge.
3 Sutcliffe S (2000) Introduction. In: Sutcliffe S, Bowman M (eds) *Beyond New Age: exploring alternative spirituality.* Edinburgh University Press, Edinburgh, pp.1–13.
4 Figl J (1991) Säkularisierung. In: Eicher P (ed.) *Neues Handbuch theologischer Grundbegriffe: Band 5.* Kösel Verlag, München, pp.84–94.
5 Hanegraaff WJ (2000) New Age religion and secularization. *Numen.* **47**: 288–312.
6 Knoblauch H (2000) Populäre Religion: Markt, Medien und die Popularisierung der Religion. *Zeitschrift für Religionswissenschaft.* **8**: 143–61.
7 Kraemer RS, Cassidy M, Schwartz SL (eds) (2001) *Religions of Star Trek.* Westview Press, Boulder, CO.
8 Porter JE, McLaren DL (eds) (1999) *Star Trek and Sacred Ground: explorations of Star Trek, religion and American culture.* SUNY Press, Albany, NY.
9 Bremmer JN (1998) 'Religion', 'ritual' and the opposition 'sacred vs. profane'. In: Graf F (ed.) *Ansichten griechischer Rituale: Geburtstags-Symposion für Walter Burkert.* Teubner, Stuttgart and Leipzig, pp.9–32.
10 Figl J (2003) Einleitung: Religionswissenschaft – Historische Aspekte, heutiges Fachverständnis und Religionsbegriff. In: Figl J (ed.) *Handbuch Religionswissenschaft.* Vandenhoeck & Rurprecht, Göttingen, pp.17–86.
11 Aulus Gellius *Noctes Atticae* [Attic nights] 4, 9, 1.

12 Cicero *De natura deorum* [About the nature of the gods] 2, 72.

13 Lactantius *Divinae Institutiones* [Divine Precepts] 4, 28, 2.

14 Herbert of Cherbury (1624) *De veritate* [About truth].

15 MacIntyre F (2004) Was religion a kinship surrogate? *Journal of the American Academy of Religion.* **72**: 653–94.

16 Eliade M (1959) *The Sacred and the Profane.* Harcourt Brace Jovanovich, New York, NY.

17 Mensching G (1959) *Die Religion: Erscheinungsformen, Strukturtypen und Lebensgesetze.* Schwab, Stuttgart.

18 Geertz C (1966) Religion as cultural system. In: Banton M (ed.) *Anthropological Approaches to the Study of Religion.* Tavistock, London, pp.1–46.

19 Smith WC (1964) *The Meaning and the End of Religion.* New American Library, New York, NY.

20 Smith JZ (1982) *Imagining Religion: from Babylon to Jonestown.* University of Chicago Press, Chicago, IL.

21 van Stietencron H (1992) Der Begriff der Religion in der Religionswissenschaft. In: Kerber W (ed.) *Der Begriff der Religion.* Kindt, München, pp.111–58.

22 Arnal WE (2000) Definition. In: Braun W, McCutcheon RT (eds) *Guide to the Study of Religion.* Cassell, London, pp.21–34.

23 Prebish CS, Keown D (2004) *Buddhism – the e-book.* Journal of Buddhist Ethics, London.

24 Hödl HG (2003) Alternative Formen des Religiösen. In: Figl J (ed.) *Handbuch Religionswissenschaft.* Vandenhoeck & Rurprecht, Göttingen, pp.485–524.

25 Oxtoby WG (2002) A personal invitation. In: Oxtoby WG (ed.) *World Religions: Western tradition* (2e). Oxford University Press, Toronto, pp.1–9.

26 Jaffee MS (2001) One god, one revelation, one people: on the symbolic structure of elective monotheism. *Journal of the American Academy of Religion.* **69**: 753–75.

27 Kuschel K-J (1995) *Abraham: sign of hope for Jews, Christians and Muslims.* Continuum, London.

28 Qur'an. *Sura.* **2**: 136.

29 Nydahl O (2004) *Wie die Dinge sind: Eine zeitgemäße Einführung in die Lehre Buddhas.* Knaur, München.

30 Scherer B (2002) *108 vragen over Boeddhisme.* Uitgeverij Milarepa, Amsterdam.

31 Assmann J (1997) *Moses the Egyptian: the memory of Egypt in Western monotheism.* Harvard University Press, Cambridge, MA.

32 Assmann J (2003) *Die Mosaische Unterscheidung oder der Preis des Monotheismus.* Carl Hanser Verlag, München.

33 Schwartz RM (1997) *The Curse of Cain. The Violent Legacy of Monotheism.* University of Chicago Press, Chicago.

34 Zenger E (2001) Was ist der Preis des Monotheismus. *Herder Korrespondenz.* **4**: 186–91.

35 Scherer B (2003) Vorwort. In: Scherer B (ed.) *Die Weltreligionen. Zentrale Themen im Vergleich.* Gütersloher Verlagshaus, Gütersloh, pp.6–7.

36 Jaspers K (1958) *Die Atombombe und die Zukunft des Menschen.* Piper, München.

37 Qur'an. *Sura.* **2**: 285 and Qur'an. *Sura.* **81**.

38 Krausen H (2003) Islam: Ethik. In: Scherer B (2003) (ed.) *Die Weltreligionen. Zentrale Themen im Vergleich.* Gütersloher Verlagshaus, Gütersloh, pp.78–9.

39 Scherer B (2001) *Buddha.* Gütersloher Verlagshaus, Gütersloh.

40 *Majjhima-Nikaya* 22.

41 Scherer B (2005) *Buddhismus: Alles, was man wissen muss.* Gütersloher Verlagshaus, Gütersloh, pp.44–5.

CHAPTER 8

An existential view: doing and being – the therapeutic relationship

Derek Mitchell

Introduction

In this chapter I will try to explore the spiritual dimension in healthcare from the point of view of existential philosophy, using primarily the work of Sartre and Heidegger and the notions of selfhood and being with others which they set out. I will try to show how these notions provide the ground for both sides of the therapeutic relationship between practitioner and patient, and how the authentic realisation of this relationship enables the self-realisation of both parties. In this way, I hope that it will become clear that what we may term the 'spiritual dimension' to healthcare is a specific manifestation of a dimension common to all human relationships. I will also look at some of the particular consequences for healthcare professionals of this necessary dimension and begin to set out how this might affect their behaviour and describe which kinds of behaviour most appropriately contribute to authentic relationships and authentic self-realisation.

Before I begin in earnest, two caveats. First I will avoid any hint that what we may term the 'spiritual dimension' has any mystical or supernatural component at all. The ground that I will be describing will, I hope, be made clear and free from obscurity and intellectual fog. Specifically, I will seek to ensure that both Sartre and Heidegger, and the tradition they represent, are immune to any mystical, magical, religious or pseudo-religious interpretation. This should not be difficult, since both were atheists; however, the complexity of their reasoning sometimes tempts commentators to retreat from explanation into vague affirmations of mysticism (or the frankly supernatural) as a means of explaining that which they do not fully understand. These kinds of suppositions are no substitute for real analysis and understanding, however difficult this may turn out to be. Second, though I will use a number of key technical philosophical terms I will try to explain these in terms of our ordinary use of language. I admit that this may not be entirely successful for the non-philosophical reader and I know at the same time it will doubtless enrage philosophical purists, but in risking pleasing no one I hope to render my thoughts intelligible to as many as possible.

Furthermore, it is worth noting that the atheism of both of these philosophers places their work firmly in the humanist camp and will provide us with a distinctly non-religious view of what is going on in healthcare. While there are also avowedly

Christian existentialists, for example Kierkergaard, for the purposes of this discussion I am confining myself to the humanist tradition in existentialism.

The chapter is divided into two main parts. In the first part I will set out the philosophical ground as follows:

- the notions of selfhood and being with others in Sartre and Heidegger
- the ideas of authenticity and self-realisation as given in this tradition
- the connectedness of being and the consequences of this analysis for individual beings.

In the second part I will focus on the following:

- the therapeutic relationship between practitioner and patient
- in the context of healthcare, the relative positions of patient and practitioner
- the specific modes of conduct that are indicated by the overall analysis.

In conclusion, I hope to show that there is a dimension in healthcare, both in the giving and the receipt, which goes beyond, and is different to, the exercise of techniques and the passive receipt of therapy, and furthermore that this is grounded in inescapable structures of selfhood that we all strive to realise. In this way I will have revealed the ontological, or underlying and very deepest, foundation of what we can call spirituality in health and social care.

Part one: the philosophers
Sartre: doing and being

In simple terms, the existential tradition proposes 'existence precedes essence', although the manifestations and development of this initial premise are many, varied and sometimes conflicting. The varieties of existential philosophy range from the avowedly Christian to the outright atheistic, and while some exponents, for example Sartre (the atheist) and Kierkergaard (a Christian), can never be brought to agreement, they share the same philosophical roots. In particular, all existentialists share the fundamental belief that we are what we do, or to put it another way, rather than each possessing a fixed essence that we then seek to realise or become, we make ourselves what we are by the choices that we make and the things that we do. Our existing comes first, and rather than explaining the things we do in terms of the way we are, the things we do make us the way we become in the first place. This starting point has many ramifications, not least that we have important choices to make about the way in which we live and the inescapable fact that, under this kind of doctrine, we are responsible not only for the choices we make but for the kind of person these choices make us into.

For the purposes of this analysis I will concentrate on what Sartre and Heidegger have to say about our relationship with others like ourselves. Although this is only part of what they are trying to say, it is the most relevant to a discussion of the relationship between healthcare practitioner and patient.

Sartre's discussion in Part III of *Being and Nothingness*[1] of the various aspects of being for Others constitutes probably the most significant part of the entire work. By describing what is there, Sartre sets out the path of possibilities available to the human actor in the world. He begins by describing the problem of the existence of

Others, sets out a few of the suggested solutions and points out their inadequacies. His methodology is made plain in 'The Reef of Solipsism'[1] (pp.223–32). He then sets out, ambitiously and ingeniously, to demonstrate the certainty of the existence of the Other in 'The Look'[1] (pp.252–302).

As is usual with Sartre, a clear thread will be discernible throughout his argument, and, despite certain flaws in the case, significant conclusions can be drawn from what he has to say.

In 'The Look', Sartre sets out his theory of the existence of Others. The first thing to notice about 'The Look' is that, although it claims simply to be a demonstration of the existence of Others, with relations between these Others discussed later, it is an intensely relational piece of philosophy. Sartre is attempting, from the point of view of the individual subject consciousness, to articulate a theory that will demonstrate that other individual conscious subjects exist beyond and independent of his own. He is thus making the ground upon which all further discussion of Others will take place and determining the fundamental relation between Others in the world.

In 'The Look' Sartre demonstrates the existence of Others through a description of certain self-evident psychological facts (unavoidable feelings, such as shame, pride and fear) which we experience, and through which we gain an immediate apprehension of the Other. Immediate apprehension is a crucial concept here – it means the apprehension of the Other not through a sensory experience (seeing, hearing, etc.) but an experience of the Other not mediated by my senses, simply welling up inside my own consciousness. The states of mind he considers are pride, shame and fear. All three operate along the same lines, so it is only necessary to give an account of one in operation.

Sartre's description of himself looking through a keyhole, suddenly surprised by footsteps coming along the corridor, is vivid. His description of the shame he feels strikes a chord. From the simple orientation of himself (as a subject) looking at the world (as an object), to the transformation of the situation by the look of an Other, and his unease under this look. Sartre claims to be saying more than simply 'I feel shame, I cannot feel such a thing alone in the world, therefore there must be Others for me to be ashamed before'. Such a deduction would be unworthy of Sartre and would miss the point of his entire project. What Sartre wishes to say is that, in shame, I actually, and immediately, experience the Other within my very being, in a way as if he were me or part of me, but it is not clear that the simple example of shame achieves all of this. Rather less emotionally compelling, and more useful philosophically, is his description of objects he sees in the park in their primary relation to him as a subject, and the way in which this description is radically reorientated when he becomes conscious of the look of the Other. As he says, 'suddenly an object has appeared which has stolen the world from me'[1] (p.255). Another subject (not me) now orientates the world and I feel this presence uncannily within my own self.

Sartre is most insistent that no space is left for inference between my own self and the Other, my apprehension of the other is immediate, 'the Other is present to me without any intermediary'[1] (p.270). This is a most intimate experience and is not the same kind of thing as the way we experience other entities in the world. This is the immediate experience of a being just like ourselves.

All sensory knowledge is subject to sceptical doubt, my senses sometimes play me false and because of this I can never be quite certain that what I think I see, hear, etc., is really there, so the only way in which Sartre can be certain of the existence of the Other is to experience the Other as a subject, not just as an object of knowledge. For this to happen a radical (and alarming) conversion must take place in which object becomes subject and subject becomes object. Sartre argues that this is what takes place in 'The Look', and that, far from being a contradiction, it is a satisfactory explanation of everyday conscious experience. Suddenly from the commanding heights of my subjectivity, seeing the world, organising its elements in my own way, I am subjected to the look of an Other and the world, including me, undergoes a reorganisation in such a way that it escapes from my control and I become an object for another subject. And 'In experiencing the look ... I experience the inapprehensible subjectivity of the Other directly and within my being'[1] (p.270). Therefore, Sartre is able to say, 'I need the Other in order to realise fully all the structures of my being'[1] (p.222).

The strongest part of Sartre's argument for the existence of Others in 'The Look' is the notion of the 'immediate apprehension of the Other'. This notion seems to capture accurately and fully the way we notice Others in the world, describing as it does the way in which Others seem to be spatially distant and yet immediately present to us. It does not matter that the two people we are talking to are six and 10 feet away respectively; both are present in exactly the same way. Thus we can say, 'it is never eyes which look at us; it is the Other as subject'[1] (p.277). By the end of 'The Look' this penetrating observation has hardened to the conclusion that, 'we have established that consciousnesses experience one another without intermediary'[1] (p.301), and Sartre is able to suggest a profound unity of being. Put in plain language, this means that my own being is set in inextricable context with that of the Other. The opposite of my self (the Other) is, as it were, the measure against which I determine my own existence.

A favourable interpretation of what Sartre says about the Other in Part III of *Being and Nothingness*[1] focuses on this unity of consciousness and the world and the way that Sartre uses the phenomena of everyday conscious experience to describe ontological structures (the fundamental building blocks of our being). Sartre uses examples of everyday experience that strike a chord with the reader. His example of looking through a keyhole and the unease we all feel when we suppose that we are discovered, and the way in which he describes our experience of the Other as a counter focus for the material world we perceive as our own, are striking and profound, yet these are simple extrapolations from everyday life. Sartre is using phenomenology in an innovative way, reminiscent of one of his earlier teachers, Martin Heidegger, to reinterpret everyday experience in a way that reveals underlying structures. Sartre's conclusions show that we are united with and not separated from each other, not as a preference or under a moral imperative, but as an inescapable fact of the way we are. I will now show how Heidegger's work improves on this position and fully develops our understanding of the inescapable relation between ourselves and others like us in the world.

Heidegger: beings in time

Martin Heidegger in his early work of 1926–1929 undermined the entire existing philosophical tradition that had come down from Descartes and changed the way we think about the world, ourselves and each other. This is set out mainly in his work *Being and Time*.[2] I will concentrate here on the part of his work relevant to our understanding of the other and show how this gives us an integrated, comprehensive and workable notion of self and the other.

Heidegger begins by rejecting the traditional idea of selfhood inherited from Descartes. Descartes famously sets the ball rolling in the Western philosophical tradition with his 'I think, therefore I am' (*cogito ergo sum*),[3] but this has already presupposed a divide between the conscious self or subject and the world 'outside', thus creating a rift which proves impossible to mend. Heidegger will propose no such division and create no such rift. Under the Cartesian conception, the individual is defined as essentially isolated not only from the world beyond but also from others like itself. It uses a model of the observing subject and represented world such that we gaze outwards at what is beyond our own self like a spectator. Heidegger correctly points out that this way of understanding ourselves and the world creates a gap between our self and everything else in the world. Once we are disconnected in this way it is impossible to reconnect ourselves and we live in this perpetual isolation. It also creates a complementary problem with the understanding of our own self in that we, as the observer, can never see ourselves. It is as if every time we try to catch a glimpse we disappear out of the corner of our own eye. It is Heidegger's primary contention that this initial division between self and not-self is fundamentally flawed and in the end sets more problems than can ever be solved. Moreover, this is just not how it really is in our everyday lives.

In common with Sartre, Heidegger begins from the existential premise 'existence precedes essence' or 'we are what we do', and he accepts that this is disconcerting in that it leaves the whole question of our nature open to question and decision. The term '*Dasein*' is central in Heidegger's work and is sometimes taken to indicate 'the self' or 'individual consciousness'; however, great care must be taken in using and understanding this term. Glendinning[4] describes it as the traditional German term for existence in general and true to the existential tradition it cannot be taken to mean the individual conscious subject or spectator. In the existential tradition, Dasein is an active self-forming notion, a doing not a being, more a verb than a noun. We are not spectators *on* the world but inescapably active participants *in* the world. We must remember that Heidegger is explicitly subverting and rejecting the whole school of philosophy which designates the self as a mere 'thing'. Dasein represents the active self-creating and self-maintaining doing.

Heidegger will conceive of no gap between ourselves and the world and constantly affirms the being in the world of Dasein. The elements we encounter are given meaning by the way that we employ them to realise the projects that we have. This is our existing. There is no spectatorial point of view and hence no problem for us in connecting with the world. But that is not all, not only do we find things in the world that we can use, we also find a world of things that are already being used by others like ourselves. Heidegger uses the term 'concern' to denote our relationship to the things we find and use. He uses the term 'solicitude' to denote the relationship we have (necessarily) to the others like ourselves that we find in the world. It is essential to remember at this point that Heidegger insists that neither of these key terms carries any moral weight, they merely denote structural or formal relationships to the two kinds of entity we encounter in the world. He is not trying to persuade us to change our behaviour towards others, just to describe how we are related.

Heidegger is trying to move beyond the kind of model of the world that had come down through the philosophical tradition since Descartes and which viewed the world as a collection of things as it were set alongside each other in the world, each waiting to be discovered and defined. Heidegger's notion of the world is as an interactive and constantly changing flux in which the projects of conscious beings change and adapt as they form and re-form through the everyday existing of human beings. This kind of thinking extends crucially to his description of our relation to others. We are in a world with others, but we are not simply alongside these others like skittles in an alley. Our relation to others is rather one of being-there-too. Our connection to other beings like ourselves is not accidental or optional but structural. He is not enjoining us to join with others or to relate sympathetically to our fellow human beings. This relationship is given and inescapable, they are part of us and we are part of them and we are just like each other, to put it another way, 'Others are encountered *environmentally*'[2] (H.155). Even when we are alone (factically or in fact) we are still the kind of being that exists essentially with others.

Paradoxically speaking we can only understand ourselves as being alone precisely because our way of being is with others. If we existed as isolated beings, the idea of 'alone' would have no meaning for us, so conversely the other can only be missing against the background of our fundamental 'Being with others'. As is usual with Heidegger's work, it is not about places and things, but about the way we go about our existing. This is emphasised further when he says:

> By 'Others' we do not mean everyone else but me – those over against whom the 'I' stands out. Rather they are those from whom, for the most part, one does not distinguish oneself – those among whom one is too.[2] (H.154)

Our unity of being with others is such that most of the time we are submerged in a world of others just like ourselves and from whom we are not distinguished.

We are now beginning to move into a position from which we can begin to see how all of this philosophy is relevant to the relationship between professional carer and client/patient. Through Heidegger's notions of concern and solicitude we can come to the relationship with new eyes, for as Heidegger says, 'Even "concern" with food and clothing, and the nursing of the sick body are forms of solicitude'[2] (H.158). This relationship is much more than any kind of social construct or moral imperative. Heidegger distinguishes two distinct forms of solicitude. Inauthentic solicitude as expressed by the 'deficient' modes (passing one another by, not 'mattering' to one another) and authentic solicitude (considerateness, forbearance) which makes the other free for their own concerns and *care*. This is another one of Heidegger's technical terms and denotes the fundamental way of being of all Dasein. Care simply means that we are all mixed up with each other and the world whether we like it or not. We cannot avoid our relationship with the world and with others because it is part of how we are made up. Dasein, as our doing, is as care, or in simpler terms Dasein can only exist as an entity involved with other entities in the world, including other Dasein. Most of the time in our everyday lives we live in the deficient modes of solicitude but this is only possible because we have the option to live authentically and because the relation of solicitude is itself inescapable.

It is left to us how we conduct ourselves towards the world and towards others, but Heidegger is making it clear that if we are to be true to ourselves at the very deepest level we should not try to avoid our interconnection with the world and with others. Authentic Dasein is being true to itself.

Dasein chooses which kind of solicitude it takes up towards others, but it cannot avoid the relationship altogether, and moreover the cost to its own being of trying to avoid, through taking up deficient modes of solicitude, will be considerable. Inauthentic Dasein does not simply deny the being of others, but in so doing denies its own authentic being because, 'As Being-with Dasein "is" essentially for the sake of Others'[2] (H.160). Conversely, Dasein, which chooses authentic modes of solicitude (considerateness, forbearance), realises its own authentic being through authentic relation to others. However, it is essential to remember that these modes of being are just that, they are not moral imperatives or any kind of injunction to act. The fundamental and structural relationship is one of being with; all subsequent modes are only possible on this foundation so that:

> 'Empathy' does not first constitute Being-with; only on the basis of Being-with does empathy become possible.[2] (H.162)

In summary, our relationship with others can be taken at two levels. First, the everyday, in which we relate to the world and others like ourselves and in which we make our choices. The second, at a much deeper level, is the way in which our very being is constructed and given to us. At this level we are fundamentally connected to the world and others such that they form that which we call our own selves. Whether we like it or not, we are submerged in the being of the world and of others and can only choose which way this is to be manifest.

Both Heidegger and Sartre make a clear case for the connectedness of being, not only connectedness with the entities we find in the world and which we use to move forward the projects which constitute our existing, but also our inescapable involvement with others like ourselves who also inhabit and use the world as we do. Heidegger is the more radical of the two in that he completely subverts the Cartesian tradition and dispenses with the notion of the isolated subject entirely, while Sartre still retains, perhaps unwillingly, vestiges of the individual subject, vestiges which ultimately make it impossible for him to free his analysis entirely from the grips of the Cartesian tradition. I will now examine how all of this abstruse theorising about the nature of self and relation to others is manifest in the day-to-day practical work that goes on between professional carers and clients and patients. I will do this first by looking briefly at some of the principles and practice of palliative care that I hope will reveal striking truths not only about this branch of healthcare, but all aspects of the care and cure of patients. I will then try to set out ways in which these truths can be realised through authentic practice in the context of a truly therapeutic relationship and a spiritual dimension to healthcare.

Part two: philosophy in practice
Palliative care and the curative impulse

My aim in this section is to show how values and principles that I believe underpin good healthcare are revealed in the practice of palliative care. These values will, not surprisingly, turn out to be a function of what is termed now as holistic care, but which have really been around for much longer than the terms we now use to describe them. They are the values of consideration and sympathy for others, respect for individuality, attending to the psychological and 'spiritual' needs of patients, and simply caring. Together they constitute what we might call the spiritual dimension of caring for others and philosophically they represent authentic being in the practice of healthcare. They are perhaps most prominent in palliative care, but I hope to show that they are also central to the delivery of care in all sectors.

Perhaps alone among the major branches of healthcare, palliative care operates without what we might call the curative impulse. This impulse to put right that which is going wrong is the major driving force in most branches of healthcare. The drive to good health and away from illness dominates any perspective on clinical practice, and while this is perhaps less evident in the treatment of chronic conditions than in acute care, the curative impulse retains a central position. Palliative care holds out no hope of ultimate cure, it is driven by quite different impulses, and has a quite different character evident in its mode of operation and the nature of its practitioners. In this, it is perhaps the most honest of all parts of care provision, because in working so closely with the fact of death it makes no attempt to deny the inevitability of death. This has the consequence that the same indicators that might be used to measure the efficacy of curatively driven treatment cannot measure the effectiveness and efficacy of palliative care. In particular, survival rates, rates of remission of chronic conditions, etc., are not applicable to an assessment of the quality of palliative care. This means that in seeking to measure quality in this area, it has been necessary to derive different and more appropriate criteria for measurement, and this in turn reveals underlying values, or the things that we think are important about palliative care, but which might also therefore be equally important to the curative branches of medicine. It is no surprise that these values and principles turn out to be very human qualities, for example empathy, understanding and respect for the individual, all of which seem to be characterised by what we may term a spiritual dimension and all of which characterise what we call holistic care. It is as if when freed from the measurement of technical operations and easily quantifiable measures, we fall back onto less tangible (and less easily measured), but more human, qualities. While I accept that the amelioration of pain in palliative care is essentially a technical discipline, I contend that this aspect of palliative care is not the defining aspect of this form of healthcare and that in its measurement it is much more subjective and less like other technical aspects of care in disciplines more directly driven by the curative impulse.

In simple terms, in most curative care contexts what we have is a situation in which where there is a possibility of cure or amelioration of the condition, or in the final instance the putting off of death to an indefinite future, these aspects of care dominate our thinking. It is only when these possibilities are removed that we are forced to consider other, more subjective, aspects of care and to consider how important they might be. The spiritual dimension is thus revealed.

It has, however, proved very difficult to develop parameters that provide a satisfactory means of measuring the quality of such subjective aspects of palliative care, and this is not really because we cannot agree on the values we want to appeal to, but more because the parameters we choose are difficult to measure. Qualitative measures such as symptom amelioration, communication, emotional support to patients and carers, treating individuals as such and with respect, the provision of information and the co-ordination of care, all present difficulties when we try to quantify them.

> The challenge is ... to find creative ways to assess client satisfaction in a manner in keeping with the holistic ... philosophy and within a process that is informed by open communication that provides every opportunity for continuous feedback from clients.[5]

Broadly speaking, we are now in the territory of quality-of-life measures, an area which is notoriously uncertain. This style is what is termed in modern parlance 'the patient-centred approach and holistic care', and from it flow the fundamental values of respect for the individuality and autonomy of others like ourselves.

In the delivery and assessment of the quality of holistic care, for example in palliative care, we measure the unmeasurable and judge success by how well the care in question lives up to our values about how we should relate to other human beings who are quite literally coming to the end of their existence. Reflecting the work of both Heidegger and Sartre, we are now considering what we might term 'relational qualities', instead of a response to the curative impulse. Patients have become people we interact with rather than objects on which we operate. In other terms, we might be said to be focusing on the spiritual dimension of healthcare rather than its technical aspects. The emphasis is more on how care is delivered as opposed to what care is delivered and this 'how' rather than any 'what' more often determines the results of delivering care. This has implications both for the patient and the healthcare professional delivering the care. The relationship between them (and with their carers and wider family members) is by no means one-way, and I will argue that an emphasis on getting the relationship between patient and practitioner right in these terms is mutually fulfilling at the deepest philosophical level.

It is really no surprise that the values and principles that are held by, and which drive, practitioners delivering holistic care are those of respect for others, the primacy of the individual, the autonomy of the patient, the satisfaction of immediate desires and needs, and similar patient-centred values. It is natural that the care of the terminally ill involves a change in priorities in relation to the patient. Treatment designed to cure becomes increasingly irrelevant as the disease progresses and other issues like friendship, company and immediate physical comfort become more and more important as the curative impulse wanes. The relationship between the professional and the patient is changed as both of their expectations as to the possible outcomes are changed. This new relationship not only more closely reflects their deeper ontological relationship, it is also the kind of relationship we would surely like to see characterise all contact between professional carers and their patients, the relationship of one human being to another. It is the foundation of holistic care.

From the work of Heidegger and Sartre we can see that we are embedded in a network of relationships with others and that these relationships themselves constitute our own selfhood. Without these relationships and outside this network we are literally nothing. We need the other to fulfil our own selves, and while in the professional carer/patient relationship there is an explicit dependence of patient on professional carer, there is also an implied and much deeper mutual dependence based on recognition of, and consequent respect for, another individual. We are structurally intertwined with the other in such a way that we become morally intertwined. Our impulse to do good for the other is founded on our inescapable ontological unity.

Returning to the debate about the measurement of quality of subjective aspects of holistic care, we can now see that measuring how well the care is being provided is a function of how well the ontological ground is represented in the more explicit behaviour of the practitioners and the responses that this elicits in patients and their carers. An attempt to disown the structural unity between human beings by failing to give recognition and respect to others will result in poor-quality care, whereas an acknowledgement of the inescapable unity of Being and its realisation in explicit behaviour produces high-quality care. At this point we can say that if the underlying ontological unity of beings constitutes a spiritual dimension, then the successful practice of holistic care constitutes the acknowledgement of this spiritual dimension. Furthermore, this recognition and its effect on practice provides a deep level of satisfaction for both client/patient and practitioner; both gain from the mutuality of the relationship and both are able to realise their authentic being-in-the-world-with-others.

Being with others and curative medicine

The example of palliative care as a non-curative care discipline shows that there is a spiritual (or philosophical) dimension to the practice of this branch of healthcare and that this dimension is revealed once the curative impulse is removed. We have also seen how good practice in palliative care exemplifies holistic care as the realisation of underlying ontological structures of being. But this form of analysis does not in any way disbar the possibility that this dimension is also present in other, curative, branches of healthcare. The curative impulse may conceal the spiritual dimension, but it is still present, or should be as part of the successful practice of all health and social care.

At a superficial level, just because in some disciplines we are able to effect a cure for the patient this should not mean that patients can be treated, for example, without respect, as diseases instead of individuals with their immediate needs and comforts disregarded or relegated to secondary importance. Instinctively we feel that patients who are properly regarded as individuals and whose needs are heard and attended to (those who are treated holistically) will 'do better' in terms of the curative process. In practical terms, they are more likely to comply with medication regimes and lifestyle changes if they are recognised and respected as individuals. Also, patients who are not treated holistically may do much worse than those who have wider needs that have been addressed. At a deeper level, any failure to respect the individuality of patients or to respect their autonomy is as likely to harm the practitioner, as it is the patient. We are driven through our being with others to regard others like ourselves in a certain manner. If we attempt to deny this and behave contrariwise, we deny not only their individuality but our own, which cannot be realised outside the network of others like ourselves. In essence, holistic care is a manifestation of our authentic relationship towards others.

The relationship between patient and practitioner is indeed therapeutic. This does not simply mean that patients get better and practitioners gain more job satisfaction; these happy circumstances are realisations of deeper structures of being that go far beyond the provision and receipt of healthcare, they address our fundamental way of being. In simple terms, the recognition of a spiritual dimension in healthcare is not only important in that it helps patients get better, but also because it enables both parties, patient and practitioner, to realise their own authentic being.

It is perhaps coincidental, or at least accidental, that this dimension only becomes apparent when we examine a discipline with no hope of cure. However, it is a lesson that is beneficial to other (curative) disciplines that cannot be exempt from, or excused, their failure to recognise this dimension as the root not only of all healthcare, but also of all human relations. Holistic care is the right way to care for all patients, not only those who are terminally ill.

Practising the virtues: realising the spiritual dimension

Having recognised the importance of the spiritual dimension to the provision of all health and social care, it now remains to see how this recognition can be realised in practice. How can we ensure that our systems of delivery of care embody the values and principles which are derived from the underlying ontological structures of being?

For this, we must turn away from familiar and traditional means of measuring the quality of care provided because these focus too strongly on areas which are indeed measurable, but which do not reflect the more fundamental relational structures between human beings. In essence, they have been more concerned with what we 'do' than anything else. In order to recognise and acknowledge the nature of being and to realise our own fundamental individuality as inescapably enmeshed with others we must change our perspective of approach and concern ourselves with how we 'are'. At the level of total systems this means replacing questions about input (resources) and outputs (results) with questions about the kind of people we want to inhabit these systems. The current focus on results (targets) obliterates consideration of the kind of people we have operating the systems. This neglect is fatal to good health and social care.

A distinctly different approach has been much promulgated in recent years through the development of Virtue Ethics[6] as an alternative to more traditional, act-focused, ethics. Virtue Ethics is distinctly agent focused and asks not whether what we are proposing to do, or have done, is right or wrong, but whether, as agents, we are virtuous in our agency. In short, are we, generally speaking, good people?

In health and social care, Virtue Ethics provides us with an opportunity to shift from the predominate focus of medical ethics on acts, to a focus on individuals. By starting to replace the question 'What is the right thing to *do*?' with the richer alternative 'What kind of person/professional ought I to *be*?', we begin to take in more morally relevant aspects found in the character of the agent and, by reducing the focus on the strict dichotomy between right and wrong, allow room for guilt, remorse, sorrow and grief as moral remainders when we have to make tragic choices. In this way, we can get away from a straightforward good/bad act dichotomy and avoid condemning those who simply make mistakes in spite of all their best efforts and intentions. Virtue Ethics allows us to look at agents as well as their acts, and opens up the moral debate by taking us away from the impasse of either/or ethics, which look only at the act. Virtue Ethics allows us to list the qualities we would like to see in our agents because it recognises that agency is crucial to action. It allows us to escape from the sterility of right/wrong act and to try to determine whether the agents are honest, trustworthy, reliable, sympathetic, etc.

In short, it enables us to make allowance for the complexity of the moral environment in which decisions are taken and the ways in which the characters of the agents affect these decisions. It is easy to see, for example, that we would want professional carers to be honest and trustworthy, compassionate and caring, sympathetic and empathetic towards their clients and patients. We value these characteristics because we believe that in any given set of circumstances professional carers who have these traits will tend to do the right thing by their patients. The problem is that as much as these qualities are desirable, they appear to be equally immeasurable. However, the measurement of the qualitative, or 'soft', aspects of health and social care practice presents a challenge not only to the tools we have available, but also to our very notion of measurability. However, it is a challenge that can be met if we are prepared to think innovatively about how we measure and how we understand measurement in terms of patients' experience. The attempts made by those assessing the quality of palliative care are instructive in this area because they represent probably the most advanced attempts so far to measure virtue.

It is essential to develop structures and systems that create virtuous agents. That is, agents (professional carers) who are honest, trustworthy, reliable, sympathetic and so on. This is based on two beliefs. The first is that health and social care is too varied and too complex to predict. This means that most of the time it is impossible to prescribe or proscribe any particular course of action as correct or incorrect and we are thrown back onto the judgement of the person providing the care. This is the most commonly stated reason as to why practice guidelines do not work. While they can provide a useful *aide memoir* and support inexperienced staff, they will never cover all eventualities.

The second belief is that experienced professionals are significantly demotivated by the over-application of quantitative measurements, and that organisations that persist in measuring themselves by their acts alone become organisations that produce statistical outcomes, rather than what might be termed 'social outcomes' (or patient health outcomes in the NHS). This belief is based on the abundant anecdotal evidence that such organisations develop systems to satisfy statistical outcomes at the expense of what might be termed 'real outcomes'. That is, they develop management solutions to the problem of providing good figures for use in league tables that have little or no regard to client or patient outcomes. These perverse incentives are not uncommon in systems that measure acts and fail to assess the virtue of their agents. This kind of behaviour by large public service institutions is understandable, if not laudable, and leads to an increasing gap between the lived experience of those people who provide and use the services, and the published figures purporting to show the performance of these institutions. This in turn destroys public confidence and trust in both the institutions and the measurement systems used to demonstrate how well they are performing. It is an explicit neglect of the spiritual dimension of health and social care and ignores many of the real needs of clients and patients.

An approach based solely on numerical target setting completely neglects any spiritual dimension to health and social care because it neglects those aspects of care which are difficult to measure and which are the most subjective. However, these are also the aspects of care which impact most closely on the relationship between client or patient and practitioner, and which are grounded in our fundamental being with others. This means that they are the aspects of care that matter most to both client or patient and practitioner. By practising the aforementioned virtues those who provide care benefit not only their clients or patients, but also themselves.

Conclusion: the therapeutic relationship

I have tried to argue from philosophical premises that what we might term 'the spiritual dimension' of health and social care is based on the ontological fact of Being-with-Others. This fundamental structure of the way that we are, is both inescapable and ultimately unavoidable, and has to be acknowledged and lived if we are to exist authentically and be true to ourselves.

In the specific context of health and social care, I have argued that the importance of relational qualities, like empathy, recognition and respect for the individuality of others, are blurred or masked in modern curative health and social care settings, but are evident in palliative care contexts, where, relieved of the curative impulse, there is a refocusing on relational qualities in measuring the efficacy of service. This shows that a more holistic approach to the provision of care and the meeting of a wide range of client or patient needs should prevail in all branches of health and social care. This, in turn, leads to the conclusion that a relationship between the client or patient and practitioner is based on qualities of mutual respect and empathy and is not only successful in achieving high standards of care and client or patient satisfaction, but at a deeper level is a realisation for all parties of authentic selfhood, and is to that extent mutually therapeutic. Furthermore, although this dimension of health and social care can go unnoticed in more explicitly curative care contexts, it is clearly of paramount importance in all areas of health and social care and is only neglected at the cost of poor treatment outcomes and the dissatisfaction and demoralisation of health and social care professionals.

Finally, I have suggested that the way in which practitioners and managers can help to ensure that the spiritual dimension of health and social care is fully recognised is to encourage virtuous agents and to concentrate more on the quality of the agents rather than their acts. What we do makes us what we are, and what we become makes us do the things we do.

References

1 Sartre J-P (1956) *Being and Nothingness – An Essay on Phenomenological Ontology* (trans. Barnes HE). Philosophical Library, New York, NY.
2 Heidegger M (1962) *Being and Time* (trans. Macquarrie J, Robinson E). Basil Blackwell, Oxford.
3 Descartes R (1986) *Meditations on First Philosophy* (trans. Cottingham J). Cambridge University Press, Cambridge.
4 Glendinning S (1998) *On Being With Others*. Routledge, London.
5 McGrath P, Wilson M (2002) Assessing hospice client satisfaction: a qualitative approach. *Progress in Palliative Care*. **10**(1).
6 Hursthouse R (1999) *On Virtue Ethics*. Oxford University Press, Oxford.

CHAPTER 9

Cultural and spiritual care

Sue Timmins

Introduction

For those who have faith, religious practice provides a source of spiritual strength when faced with difficult circumstances or ill health. In a multicultural population, the provision of care needs to be sensitive to the consequent diversity of religious practice and cultural identity. This chapter considers how raising the awareness of professional carers, combined with the development of an ethos of client/patient empowerment, provides the means of moving towards care which recognises multi-faith needs. Diet, ritual, physical examination, competing needs, interpretation of language and issues relating to care of the dying are each considered in turn.

The multicultural population

The range of patients and clients requiring care in the UK now embraces multicultural populations as the norm, and as a result, healthcare provision needs to be sensitive to increased diversity. This need was first outlined in the White Paper *The New NHS: modern, dependable,*[1] which stated that healthcare should be '...a personal service, responsive to the needs of individual patients...'.

Cultural issues reflect both domestic and international backgrounds and lifestyles. Within the UK, for example, there could be a world of difference in the outlook on life between a single black mother in a northern inner-city deprived area, surviving on state benefits, and a white middle-class retired Midlands widower with his own house, a good pension and a network of employed children who care for his welfare.

Those who are less culturally aware may not always draw the distinction between cultural practices and religious obligations, and consequently, there may be un-certainty as to whether the adherence to a particular practice has its roots in religious duties or in influence from the patient's cultural background.

Adherences to religious practices can vary greatly. While the basic concepts of a religion will remain inherently the same wherever it is practised, the way in which an individual may demonstrate their beliefs may vary. For example, some Muslims will pray five times a day, and others, although their faith is otherwise strong, will not. Similarly, some Christians go to church every Sunday, or more frequently, and others will go less often, or not at all. Human nature is such that an individual's requirements are often adapted to meet their own circumstances or consciences. It must be recognised by those providing care that cultural and religious practices cannot be compartmentalised, and that the adherence to and adoption of both cultural and religious norms may be different in individual patients. Swinton[2] observed that assumptions must not be made that the culture and religion of a person's country of origin will necessarily influence, to the same degree, the habits and beliefs of all people sharing that origin.

It must also be acknowledged that there are many people indigenous to the UK who have converted from the State faith of Christianity to other religions, and their needs must be recognised equally alongside those of the immigrant population.

Within the UK, both indigenous and immigrant patients and clients may still lack awareness of their right to ask for clarification about the treatments and medications they are given. Maslow[3] identified the baseline of human requirements as 'safety', and there is no doubt that, particularly in times of stress and ill health, the basic human need is to return to the familiar. For example, many people in normal daily life want to go home if they are unwell, because everything there is recognisable, comforting and close at hand. In the same way, being enabled to continue to participate in religious and cultural practices while undergoing healthcare interventions can assist the client's/patient's feeling of spiritual fulfilment, even while still remaining ill or under stress. In times of difficulty and poor health, some clients/patients may feel that they are among professionals who are caring but not understanding of their personal circumstances, and so may feel a desperate requirement for familiar reminders and reassurances, or for words that will bring succour and peace. There is great satisfaction in knowing that some aspects of life do not have to change despite the circumstances in which the individuals find themselves. The recognition that professional carers acknowledge these needs will also give comfort and reassurance to the patient's relatives and carers. Promoting the spiritual wellbeing of their client/patient may enable them to feel more at ease and more responsive to the healthcare professionals' interventions.

Raising awareness in health and social care

In order to respond appropriately to the cultural and religious needs of their patients and clients, all health and social care professionals must have a broad understanding of those needs. Many health authorities have produced documentation for their staff on cultural and religious awareness. Examples of these are the local guides produced by Bath Health Promotion Unit[4] and Lothian Racial Equality Council,[5] as well as publications for a wider audience.[6] Recent European Union directives[7] require compliance from member states in ensuring equal opportunity and ease of access to health and social care for all patients and clients, irrespective of background and religious conviction.

Hopkins and Bahl[8] suggest that an awareness of the patient's or client's culture can provide the health professional with a deeper insight into their behaviour in illness, and thus improve the quality of care provided. Professional carers should recognise that patients and clients from minority groups may have different concepts about health and illness, as well as different expectations from consultations and care delivery. This awareness will help carers to gain the confidence of their patients, and those in their care are more likely to comply with advice and treatment.

Battacharyya[9] supports the theory that crises in health and similar situations arouse responses which prompt individuals to seek solutions often learned in their childhood development. He recognises that culture and language become paramount to the patient under stress, and that the therapist or carer can influence the success of episodes of care by communicating with the patient at an appropriate level, and in an empathetic manner. Similarly, Lau[10] endorsed a relationship between patient and therapist in which the importance of familiar rituals and practices could be acknowledged. Lau felt that this approach would counteract the perception that Western-trained doctors are preoccupied with medical procedures. Lack of empathy might inadvertently motivate patients from differing cultural backgrounds to seek traditional, or alternative, medicines from practitioners within their own cultural groups.

The value of staff training was exemplified by Prime,[11] who describes how anti-racist training could inform social work staff of how their own prejudices might affect their feelings and attitudes towards their clients. Similar training might be equally beneficial to healthcare professionals. Without a broad understanding of the issues encountered by patients from backgrounds and cultures very different from their own experience, professional carers may inadvertently create barriers of misunderstanding or prejudice, which could adversely affect healthcare provision.

There are particular times when the diversity of needs of the individual becomes more apparent, for example at birth and death. Cultural or religious requirements and practices may influence the way in which the care of the newborn or dying person is managed. Culturally sensitive care should permeate all aspects of health provision throughout the patient's life, whether it is given in the community or acute setting, or in the private or voluntary sectors. Professional carers need to recognise and value the differences in cultural and religious perceptions. Over a decade ago, McAvoy and Donaldson[12] highlighted the importance of training, not only for the clinical team, but for all the members of the wider team, to ensure that all personnel with patient contact are culturally aware. Their reference to non-clinical staff must extend to healthcare assistants, clerical personnel, housekeeping and portering staff, to name but a few.

The Government White Paper *The Health of the Nation*[13] highlighted the importance of addressing the health needs of people from ethnic minorities, and heralded the acknowledgement that some areas of the NHS may have been slow to respond to the needs of minority groups. Subsequent work[14] makes specific reference to the ethnic minority population in the UK, and to the morbidity and mortality patterns of specific groups within that population. Subsequent Government documents have built on these foundations; for example, the White Paper *The New NHS: modern, dependable*[1] stated clearly the intention that everyone in the nation shall have:

> ...fair access to health services in relation to people's needs, irrespective of geography, class, ethnicity, age or sex. For example, ensuring that black and minority ethnic groups are not disadvantaged in terms of access to service. (Section 8, para 5.ii)

However, in practice, clients'/patients' perceptions of the ideal model of a sensitive and responsive healthcare service may still be quite different from this ideal. Neile[15] (quoting[16]) considered that:

> ...the NHS remains essentially geared to the attitudes, priorities and expectations of the majority population, which is considered white, middle class, and nominally Christian. (pp.31–2)

The need to raise healthcare professionals' awareness of diversity was clearly highlighted in the 1990s. However, near the end of that decade, Ahmed (cited[17]) pointed out that healthcare provision in the UK was still based on Western medical models, which did not reflect the beliefs, values and attitudes to health held by minority ethnic communities. This statement can be challenged by many who now disagree with it, but there remains a distinct possibility that those healthcare professionals who have only a limited understanding of the cultural and religious needs of their patients, either through lack of training or lack of exposure, may be delivering a service which is said to be fair, caring and undiscriminating to all, but which, in fact, fails to recognise or allow for the specific needs of individual patients.

Neile[15] comments that 'a service is only relevant if it caters for the perceived needs of the population which is using it' (p.118), and this does mean that cultural awareness and an understanding of religious norms should be part of the core of today's healthcare delivery for all patients.

There remain areas of the country where exposure to minority patients is infrequent, and where the levels of awareness and opportunity to demonstrate cultural and religious sensitivity may be limited. Consequently, the need to deliver a culturally sensitive service is less pronounced. This is not to say that the healthcare delivered in those areas is of any less high standard – only that, when such an opportunity does arise, the specific cultural and religious needs of the individual patients may be less easily recognised and met.

Narayanasamy's ACCESS model[18] (Table 9.1) is a valuable tool to assist in the application of knowledge of cultural and religious variances to individual patients, and also to encourage the development of personal cultural and religious awareness by those in health and social care. This ACCESS model outlines a strategy that is helpful in promoting the provision of sensitive care.[18] Professional carers do not have to agree personally with, or comply with, a patient's cultural or religious practices, but need to set aside any reservations or prejudices while delivering care to that patient. They also need to acknowledge those practices and beliefs as having validity and importance to the individual patient.

Table 9.1   The ACCESS model[18]

Assessment	Focus on cultural aspect of patient's lifestyle, health beliefs, and health practices
Communication	Be aware of variations in verbal and non-verbal responses
Cultural negotiation and compromise	Become more aware of aspects of other people's cultures, and more understanding of their views and their explanations of their problems
Establish respect and rapport	Develop a therapeutic relationship which portrays genuine respect for patients' cultural beliefs and values
Sensitivity	Deliver diverse, culturally sensitive care to culturally diverse patients
Safety	Enable patients to derive a sense of safety

This tool can also be used as an integral part of the overall assessment of patients' spiritual needs, and therefore should be reflected in the use of other tools, e.g. Govier[19] and Ross.[20]

Empowering the patient

The Parekh Report[21] examined all aspects of the needs of ethnic minorities, including healthcare. It endorsed the need for the NHS and independent care providers to ensure that the ethnic minority communities actually understood the services on offer, and cited the case of the cervical screening service in east London. Historically, women from the Asian subcontinent had not accessed this service,[22] but once it was explained to them using language and terminology they could understand, they embraced it and supported it enthusiastically. Cultural sensitivity about these processes led to a successful outcome, with the service meeting the needs of the local community, and a consequent improvement in their overall wellbeing.

In general, clinical staff will find that their patients are happy to discuss their specific requirements, once they realise that their needs will be addressed sensitively. It may be that all needs identified cannot be fulfilled, for instance not every healthcare site will have a multi-faith prayer room, but it will help the patient enormously to know that their priorities are acknowledged and that those caring for them will do all they can to support them.

Dietary issues

Client/patient dietary requirements may be influenced by cultural and/or religious views. Many do not realise that inpatient units are required to be equipped to provide menus which are compliant with, among others, kosher and halal food laws. These are the religious requirements for meat provision for persons following the Jewish and Islamic (Muslim) faiths respectively; animals and poultry are slaughtered in accordance with religious laws, with the name of God being invoked at the time of death, and persons of those faiths are prohibited from eating meat and poultry slaughtered in any other manner. Where they are uncertain about the origin of meat, Jewish and Muslim clients/patients may prefer a vegetarian diet. In all instances where patients do not wish to eat meat, vegetarian options should be available. It may be that clients/patients will in fact eat whatever is proffered, even if they would not eat it at home. They may do this to please the healthcare professional, but may carry subsequent unrequited feelings of guilt because they have contravened their religious laws. This guilt will affect their general feeling of wellbeing until (or if) it can be expunged by prayer or ritual. These situations are easily prevented by a sensitive approach by the inpatient unit's hotel services staff, and by recognising the need for patient choice of menu.

In relation to the subject of diet, it is important that professional carers are aware that, for Muslim clients/patients, the right hand is 'clean' and used for eating, but the left hand is 'dirty' and used for cleaning the body. The issue of laterality also arises when caring for hemiplegic Muslim patients, where the patient's inability to use the appropriate hand may cause distress, and will require sensitive negotiation by professional carers.[23]

The dietary requirements of those following religions other than Christianity have implications reaching beyond catering, which must be recognised. Dietary constraints also apply to medication, and where medication contains substances that are forbidden, alternatives should be explored. A prime example of this has been the provision of medication for diabetes, where either pork- or beef-based insulin was used before human equivalents were available. Consumption of products containing pork and beef are forbidden to Muslims and Jews, and Hindus respectively. Similarly, many capsules are formulated with gelatin, which is frequently pork-based. Recognition must also be given to those liquid medications and treatments which have an alcohol base, and these should be avoided when caring for those patients for whom alcohol is a forbidden substance.[6,24]

The religious calendars followed by patients from a non-Christian background should also be taken into consideration, in particular in those faiths where fasting forms a vital part of obligatory or voluntary rituals. During times of fast, strict adherents may refuse to take oral medication in either solid or liquid form, and discussion will have to take place with individual clients/patients as to whether the administration of intravenous or transdermal medications at these times is an acceptable alternative.[25,26] It should be borne in mind that the ill Muslim is exempted from fasting, but may still elect to do so as a personal decision.

Patients' failure to take medication as instructed (referred to as non-compliance or, more recently, non-concordance) is a recognised problem in healthcare. Non-compliance in clients/patients from minority ethnic or religious backgrounds has not been specifically researched, but there are a number of possible reasons for this (Box 9.1).

Box 9.1   Potential reasons for non-compliance

- In instances where the patient is from a non-English-speaking background, it may simply be that the patient (and/or their carer) has not understood the dispenser's instructions, or cannot read or translate the dispensing instructions on the packaging.
- If the patient is from a background with heavy reliance on traditional or herbal medication, pharmaceutical interventions may be unfamiliar and treated with suspicion unless their efficacy is fully understood.
- The patient may be fully aware of the composition of the medication and recognise that it contains forbidden components, and may make a deliberate decision not to comply, without understanding that acceptable alternatives might be available if they notify healthcare staff about their concerns.
- The patient may be fasting, either voluntarily or as an obligation, and may, for instance, be taking oral medication only during the hours of darkness when ingestion by mouth is permitted.

An awareness of potential reasons for client/patient non-compliance by health professionals, together with supportive remedial action such as the offering of alternatives, will contribute to patients' overall spiritual and physical wellbeing.

Religious and cultural requirements

Matters specific to individual religious practices must be taken into account. For example, Sikhism requires that its followers adhere to the carrying of the '5 Ks' about their person.[6] The healthcare professional may expect to find a Sikh patient with the following:

- uncut hair (kesh)
- carrying about their person a comb (kangha)
- and a symbolic dagger (kirpari)
- wearing a steel bangle (kara)
- and symbolic shorts (kaccha).

It is important to acknowledge a Sikh patient's need to continue to wear or carry these items when in healthcare settings. Similarly, significant items may be worn or carried by people of other faiths at different times in their lives, or throughout life, and healthcare professionals should familiarise themselves with these practices.

Physical examination

Some religious cultures may have strict requirements about being examined, intimately or more generally, by persons of the opposite sex.[6,23] For instance, in daily life, strict Muslim women will cover their entire body when in public, generally only exposing the face, hands and feet, but even these body parts may be covered in some strict cultural interpretations. They may wish not to expose their body to any man other than their husband, and similar restrictions will apply to men, who may wish to keep the area from waist to knee covered. In these circumstances, patients may find it reassuring to know that they can request consultation with a professional of their own sex. However, many faiths and cultures do acknowledge that some of their required practices can be set aside should it be absolutely essential in the interests of patient care. This decision should be made by the individual where possible, and not generally assumed to be acceptable to all.

Professional carers need to balance meeting the diverse needs of minority groups with those of the majority population. For instance, the perception that asylum seekers are given special treatment has been deeply resented in certain parts of the country, particularly where special services have been set up for them.[27] Similarly, in an institutional setting, patients might believe that others are receiving preferential treatment if they are given different menus, or having their wish to pray in private recognised. While these opportunities should be available to all patients on request, intolerance born of misunderstanding can arise. Professionals may also make assumptions and be unaware of their own prejudices, which could result in insensitivity at times like this. A positive attitude, with an underlying knowledge and understanding of how religious practices need to be accommodated in health and social care settings, is needed in order to be able to provide a balanced and sensitive service to all those needing care.

Language and interpretation

Similar challenges are posed when considering interpretation facilities, and chaperoning. Patients with a limited grasp of English may present at consultations with their families, and use a young child or male relative for interpretation. This practice is recognised as causing problems in the transmission of information.[28] In these circumstances there is no assurance that the information is being translated and relayed accurately, and also, the family interpreter may have personal embarrassments or prejudices which influence the consultation. The child may have difficulty in understanding the medical situation and terminology, and the parent may be embarrassed in front of the child. Similarly, male members of the family may not wish to discuss health matters with or in the presence of clinical personnel, particularly if these are gynaecological or otherwise sexual in nature. For similar reasons, it is inappropriate for family members to request to chaperone patients, as chaperoning activities must be undertaken by a trained healthcare professional, so that they can recognise if inappropriate activities are taking place. The Ayling Report[29] was specific on this point. For the protection of both patient and clinician, an untrained chaperone may not understand if either the clinician's or the patient's actions or verbal comments are inappropriate for the procedure being undertaken. Cultural sensitivity at this time will be reassuring and supportive to the patient. Sometimes, very small alterations in the examination practices of individuals, such as using separate towels for drying the hands after touching the patient below and above the waist, will demonstrate sensitivity.

In addition to practices relating to religious observations, the healthcare professional needs to have a basic awareness of the way in which cultural influences and ethnic origin can affect consultations, and the presentation of symptoms. For example, many first-generation immigrants of Afro-Caribbean origin believe that it is disrespectful to make eye contact with someone who they consider to be their superior; in the consultation, they may believe that they should defer to the healthcare professional and thus may not look directly at them. This could be interpreted as lack of interest or insolence by the uninformed practitioner, but is far from the case.

Neile[15] cites a case of a pregnant Asian patient who did not attend a regular antenatal class, since at her first visit the patient found that what was being taught differed widely from the cultural norm of her matriarchal experience in her home country. She also refers to the fact that in some cultures, post-partum women do not leave their homes for 40 days after childbirth, and similar isolationist practices can be followed when women and girls are menstruating. A culturally uninformed health visitor suggesting to an Asian mother that her baby should be weaned onto proprietary jars of baby food may cause consternation, since for generations the babies in that family have been weaned on mild curries, preparing them for their future spicy adult menu. As cultural practices inform the whole of a patient's lifestyle, a more sensitive awareness, in this case, of dietary need, would instil greater confidence in healthcare provision as well as contributing to overall well-being.

Cultural and religious practice in terminal care

At the end of life, the needs of the patient and their family in terminal care are vital to their peace of mind. Many religious and cultural groups will have very specific rituals and formalities which they will wish to follow at this time, and the sensitive healthcare professional will be able to facilitate these. Family members and religious elders may wish to participate in these rituals, which ensure the successful transition of the dying person into the afterlife, or secure the wellbeing of their soul, and will give much comfort to those left behind (*see* Appendix).

Many faiths prefer that the bodies of their dead are washed and covered in accordance with their traditions, some of which will be that family members would like to be consulted and, if possible, involved in the laying out of the deceased. Family members or a representative of the religion may wish to remain with the body at all times immediately after death and possibly for the following 24 hours.

For both Jews and Muslims, cremation is not desirable, and burial ideally takes place within 24 hours. Hindus and Sikhs desire cremation within a similar time-scale. This can present problems if a postmortem is required, as this is not always immediately practical, and certification of death has to take place in accordance with due legal procedure. It is important that the healthcare professional determines from family or carers the processes which they would ideally wish to be followed, and facilitates these where possible.

However, sensitivity to other patients in the same setting must also be taken into consideration. For example, certain religious sects and cultures (such as the Shia Muslims from Iran) tend to mourn loudly over the deceased, which is unusual in the indigenous UK culture. In an inpatient unit, this might be disturbing to other patients or their families. Sensitivity and tolerance are needed to enable rituals and practices to be followed as far as possible, without causing distress to others who are ill.

An appreciation of the likely requests that might be received from members of different religious and cultural groups when one of their members dies will be a considerable asset to those involved in the delivery of care at this time.

Conclusion

It is integral to the success of healthcare interventions that those delivering care are culturally aware, and demonstrate that awareness in their interactions with their patients, clients, and their families and carers. Patients may earnestly desire to cling to familiar religious and cultural practices with which they feel comfortable, and which give them a feeling of security and peace of mind. This may be particularly evident in times of sickness and stress, when they may be in unfamiliar environments. Where, due to individual circumstances, compromises between the patient's wishes and the practicalities of the care environment have to be negotiated, options should be presented in a sensitive and reassuring manner. Acknowledgement and support of cultural and religious needs by health and social care professionals contribute to the spiritual wellbeing of those in their care.

References

1   Secretary of State for Health (1997) *The New NHS: modern, dependable*. HMSO, London.
2   Swinton J (2001) *Spirituality and Mental Health Care: rediscovering a 'forgotten' dimension*. Jessica Kingsley Publishers, London.
3   Maslow A (1987) *Motivation and Personality* (3e). HarperCollins, London.
4   Bath Health Promotion Unit (1996) *Respect for Privacy, Dignity, and Religious and Cultural Beliefs*. Bath HPU, Bath.
5   Lothian Racial Equality Council (1992) *Religions and Cultures – a guide to patients' beliefs and customs for health service staff*. Lothian REC, Edinburgh.
6   Timmins S (2003) *Patients' Cultural and Religious Issues: a guide for primary care*. Aeneas Press, Chichester.
7   www.eoc.org.uk/EOCeng/EOCs/Legislation/towardsequalityanddiversity: (website accessed 1 March 2005).
8   Hopkins A, Bahl V (1993) *Access to Health Care for People from Black and Ethnic Minorities*. Royal College of Physicians, London.
9   Battacharyya A (2005) *Good Communication: key to transcultural therapies*. www.priory.com/psych/astrange.htm (website accessed 7 March 2005).
10 Lau BWK (1991) What is scientific medicine? In: Squires AJ (ed.) *Multicultural Health Care and Rehabilitation for Older People*. Edward Arnold, Sevenoaks.
11 Prime R (1991) Social work with minority ethnic elders. In: Squires AJ (ed.) *Multicultural Health Care and Rehabilitation for Older People*. Edward Arnold, Sevenoaks.
12 McAvoy BR, Donaldson LJ (eds) (1990) *Health Care for Asians*. Oxford University Press, Oxford.
13 Secretary of State for Health (1992) *The Health of the Nation*. Her Majesty's Stationery Office, London.
14 Balarajan R, Raleigh VS (1993) *The Health of the Nation: ethnicity and health, a guide for the NHS*. Department of Health, London.
15 Neile E (1997) Control for black and ethnic minority women; a meaningless pursuit. In: Kirkham MJ, Perkins ER (eds) *Reflections on Midwifery*. Ballière Tindall, London.
16 Weller B (1991) Nursing in a multicultural world. *Nursing Standard*. **5**(30): 31–2 .
17 Rawaf S, Bahl V (eds) (1998) *Assessing Health Needs of People from Ethnic Minority Groups*. Royal College of Physicians and The Faculty of Public Health Medicine, London, pp.324, 326.
18 Narayanasamy A (1999) The ACCESS Model: a transcultural nursing practice framework. *Nurse Education Today*. **19**: 274–85 (reproduced with permission of Elsevier Ltd).
19 Govier I (2000) Spiritual care in nursing: a systematic approach. *Nursing Standard*. **14**(17): 32–6.
20 Ross LA (1998) The nurse's role in spiritual care. In: Cobb M, Robshaw V (eds) *The Spiritual Challenge of Health Care*. Churchill Livingstone, Edinburgh.
21 Parekh B (2000) *The Future of Multi-Ethnic Britain*. Profile Books, London.
22 Naish J, Brown J, Denton B (1994) Intercultural consultations: investigation of factors that deter non-English speaking women from attending their general practitioners for cervical screening. *BMJ*. **309**(6962): 1126–8.
23 Hume C (1991) Introducing treatment and selection of media. In: Squires AJ (ed.) *Multicultural Health Care and Rehabilitation for Older People*. Edward Arnold, Sevenoaks.
24 Blenkinsop A, Panton R, Partop I (1991) Ethnic minority elders and the pharmacy. In: Squires AJ (ed.) *Multicultural Health Care and Rehabilitation for Older People*. Edward Arnold, Sevenoaks.
25 www.ethnicityonline.net/islam_diet: (website accessed 1 March 2005).
26 www.bbc.co.uk/religion/religions/islam/features/ramadan/health~: (website accessed 1 March 2005).
27 www.wsws.org/articles/1999/aug199/~ (website accessed 1 March 2005).
28 Henley A (1979) *Asian Patients in Hospital and at Home*. Tunbridge Wells, Pitman Medical.
29 Ayling Report (2004) *Committee of Enquiry – independent investigation into how the NHS handled allegations about the conduct of Clifford Ayling*. Department of Health, London.

Creative therapy

CHAPTER 10

Therapy and wellbeing

Bons Voors

Introduction

This chapter considers the work of the Blackthorn Trust, a health and rehabilitation centre within a National Health Service (NHS) general practitioner (GP) surgery. Blackthorn exemplifies a spiritual approach to care provision that is underpinned by the philosophy of Rudolf Steiner. An overview of anthroposophical medicine is given, followed by a description of the establishment of the Blackthorn community. This is followed by examples of therapy offered to patients at Blackthorn.

Anthroposophy; a short introduction to the insights of Rudolf Steiner

The word 'anthroposophy' comes from the Greek *anthropos*, man, and *sophia*, wisdom, meaning 'the wisdom of our humanity'. Rudolf Steiner, an Austrian philosopher and scientist (1861–1925), shared his insights on anthroposophy in a great number of books[1] and many lectures during the first quarter of the twentieth century. From childhood, Rudolf Steiner was aware of an ability to perceive the spiritual realities that lie hidden behind the material world. He trained in mathematics, physics and chemistry in Vienna and went on to edit Goethe's complete scientific works. His own work has found practical application in the renewal of medicine, education, agriculture, community life and within the various forms of art.

- *Education* in Waldorf Schools emphasises developing the child's whole spectrum of aptitudes and ability to fully be themselves. The curriculum is based on *'head, heart and the hands'* of pupils, and so highlights the emotional and intellectual development of the child alongside practical activity. Steiner's style of education also acknowledges the value of art in learning by its strong emphasis on an artistic approach in all subjects.
- *Biodynamic agriculture* aims to produce healthy and organic food by using methods that serve the earth, the plant and mineral kingdoms, as well as providing nutrition for man.
- *Community life* was developed in the Camphill Movement. Since 1945 this has brought about a meaningful way of living and working together for mentally and physically handicapped children and adults. By developing a new social pedagogy, a way of life was created which addresses the particular demands of

people with special needs. Staff and their families, young co-workers and the special needs people live and join together in meaningful work, education, and a rich life of festivals and artistic creativity.
- In the *arts*, Rudolf Steiner brought a renewing impulse to the fields of architecture, painting, sculpture, eurythmy (which is a form of movement), speech and music.[2]

Not only was Steiner a scientist and philosopher, but he also had insights into the invisible or supersensible world. He claimed that this path of 'spiritual science' was open to everyone and gave many indications of how to develop one's thinking and faculties to perceive the sense world at a deeper level.

Basic to all these fields are his concepts of the developing human being within a world of evolution where the macrocosmos of the universe and the microcosmos of man are completely interlinked. The work of Rudolf Steiner, while fully recognising advances in natural science, sought to extend its boundaries with a 'Science of Spirit'. His research explored the unique nature and potential of the human being and clarified how, in health and illness, the individual human spirit, ego and soul interact within the body.

Anthroposophical medicines and remedies

Anthroposophical medicines make use of man's relationship with and are prepared from mineral, plant and animal substances. The medicines were originally developed in the 1920s as an extension to the conventional medicines available. They exist in many different forms, such as tablets, dilutions, injections, ointments, oils, powders, suppositories and lotions. Traditional pharmaceutical and homeopathic techniques are used in a specifically anthroposophical way. The products range from over-the-counter remedies to prescription-only medicines and are manufactured using stringent quality controls and modern pharmaceutical technology. Wherever possible, the plants and herbs, are grown by the manufacturers themselves, and are therefore free from artificial fertilisers or pesticides. To ensure the purest ingredients, Steiner's organic method of cultivation, called biodynamic agriculture, is used. Many of the medicines and remedies are developed for specific illnesses and disorders. The most well-known of these are Viscum preparations, which are based on mistletoe (*Viscum album*) and used to stimulate the immune system, particularly for treatment of cancer.[3]

Anthroposophical therapies

Anthroposophical therapies address human developmental needs in illness through the arts. Arts are connected to the divine and the creative in man. In order to test the validity of Rudolf Steiner's work and use it to build on conventional knowledge, the anthroposophical doctor and therapist have to learn to broaden and strengthen their thinking, perception and experience. This is achieved through training that includes meditative exercises and methods of observation of the natural world. The principal aim of the anthroposophical approach is to derive ways of encouraging patients to actively engage in their own treatment and rehabilitation. Illness is seen not as just a threat, but as an important and sometimes necessary challenge, giving stimulus to self-development. The individual may thereby find new purpose in their life and better control of their destiny.[4] The main therapies used to enhance this process are rhythmical massage, eurythmy, biographical counselling, art therapy and music.

Body, soul and spirit

An important aspect in anthroposophical medicine is the understanding of how body, soul and spirit interact in health and illness, and which part needs to be addressed or strengthened either through medicaments or therapy. The different therapies have also a very specific role to play in this respect.

In anthroposophical medicine, the meaning of the words 'body', 'soul' and 'spirit' are as follows:[4]

- **Spirit** or **ego** represents man's unique, eternal and essentially moral self. Through the ego, man accomplishes his everyday and higher aims on earth. The human ego unfolds through the process of education and growing up. It strengthens itself by taking on and mastering or suffering life's challenges and obstacles. It is responsible for individual human development and enables one to take charge of one's life and some control over one's destiny.
- **Soul** endows the individual with character and a wide range of abilities. The soul's activities may be divided into *three spheres*, each of which arises within and is coordinated by its own bodily system. The nervous system provides the basis for sense perception and *thinking*. The senses allow us to appreciate the world we live in. Thinking brings intelligence to decision making and gives one capacity to further one's self-knowledge and development. Organs with a predominantly rhythmical function, notably breathing and circulation, create and sustain a rich life of *feeling*. Incoming perceptions stimulate imagination, rouse desires and establish moods, which in turn influence what we decide to do and how we set about it. The body's metabolism and limbs give power and expression to *the will* through which the individual makes himself felt by his deeds.
- **Body** refers to the complex living instrument that the individual inhabits and makes use of to carry out all his daily tasks. The body has two aspects: a physical part, whose substances take their origin from the mineral world, and an etheric part, whose processes infuse the mineral substance and bring it into life. These processes are guided by the ego and soul in holding the delicate balance between processes that build the body up and processes that break it down, thereby maintaining the constancy of form.

This outline barely begins to summarise Steiner's far-reaching insights of anthroposophical medicine that he developed with a Dutch doctor, Ita Wegman. Greater detail on this subject is found in the writings of Evans and Rodger[5] and Douch.[3]

Anthroposophical therapy in a community setting

The Blackthorn Trust is a health and rehabilitation centre whose work is inspired by Rudolf Steiner. Set up 20 years ago to serve the seriously and chronically ill, it was a small initiative started in a NHS GP surgery. However, as the workload increased, the surgery premises became too cramped. Following an incredible fundraising drive by staff and patients to gather the means of providing a purpose-designed building, Blackthorn was transferred to a new home, The Blackthorn Medical Centre. Rudolf Steiner's ideas on architecture gave the new building form and orientation. The building was designed using form and colour to provide an environment that serves the healing process of the patient. Equally, it was to be a space where festivals could be celebrated, and small, intimate concerts and talks given as part of a cultural and educational healing activity. At the same time NHS and social service funds for patients with long-term mental health conditions provided the means for acquiring a walled, derelict garden adjacent to the new building.

From involving just one art therapist, working one day a week with so-called 'heart-sink' patients (who make the doctor's 'heart sink' because of their frequent visits without there being, or seeming to be, any further options or solutions available for them), Blackthorn has become a flourishing enterprise offering five forms of therapy: art, music, rhythmical massage, counselling and curative eurythmy. These provide the doctors with different options for helping their patients, particularly those who are very seriously ill and those with long-term chronic conditions. Doctors and therapists work as a team after the initial referral of the patient by the doctor to one or more therapists. Steiner's ideas are used as a hypothesis to be worked with, tested and explored. The team studies together and shares insights about the patient. The patient is aware that he or she plays a vital role in the process of healing. Doctor and therapist encircle the patient with support and appropriate challenges, but the patient is the key player.

One of the premises that underpin this approach to care is that these therapies should be available to those who need them regardless of their means; patients are not expected to pay for treatment. Funding of the Trust comes from various means, but does include fundraising activity by patients who wish to give something back to the Trust. In fact, participating in fundraising activities has become part of the process of healing for some patients, as well as contributing to community building. In this way, people are not simply ill and get their individual treatment, but help each other and become part of a community where all manner of activities take place, such as workshops, concerts and fairs.

The Trust shop can provide patients with a protected place where they can get involved and feel of value again in serving others. All these opportunities form part of 'treatment' on the road to wellbeing. So often, serious illness, depression and loneliness make people very isolated. They lose confidence, are unable to work and their relationship with the world can be seriously affected. Activities in Blackthorn Garden include a small vegetarian café with a bakery, organic gardens, greenhouses and a 'secret garden', where patients with mental health problems can work and develop. The formula is simple and brilliant. Mix illness and health together and address the healthy aspect of every human being. This means that patients, plus volunteers, and the public who come for a delicious lunch in the café or to buy fresh bread from the bakery or a plant or two from the shop, form a healthy community – or perhaps one that is better described as – a *health-giving* community, for workers and visitors alike.

So, fundamentally, Blackthorn utilises two sources of therapy to promote healing. First, the one-to-one therapeutic work by doctors and therapists (although this is augmented by group work as well), for example artistic therapies, painting, sculpture, music and eurythmy, as well as massage and biographical counselling. The other is rehabilitation through work and engagement in the Blackthorn Garden, the craft groups, the land and the café, with its main emphasis on healing in *community life*. Successful therapy has resulted in a third type of support being developed. As life at Blackthorn can become too comfortable for patients, a programme was created to help people move on, back into the wider world. Workways is a programme for Trust patients and also for people from outside the Trust who have been out of work for a long time. It provides support and help for patients to find either paid or voluntary work or enter into educational programmes. The educational element for patients in the garden – or co-workers as they are called – has steadily increased to help people grow, learn new skills and build confidence.

Over time, Blackthorn has developed into a setting where a host of possible therapeutic and educational options are available to address the needs of the individual who is unwell. The key is not to address just the patient's illness but the individual's needs on their journey to becoming whole.

Biographical counselling, an example of individual therapy

Biographical counselling relates to the view that our biography is our own life story. In reality, people, clients or patients often have great difficulty with parts of their life story. They would like to tear out some of the pages of their autobiography, as often it is very difficult to accept loss of work, bereavement, the onset of long-term or terminal illness. So often the threads of destiny seem to have become so entangled, that all sense of meaning and purpose is lost. Within the biographical counselling setting the therapist accompanies the client to help them own their own life story with all the joyful and painful parts included. The task at hand is not so much solving 'the problem' the patient presents (although that may be very helpful as well), but getting a sense of where this issue has a place in the totality of the individual's life; of what was before and what comes next. A joint exploration is undertaken to understand how an event, crisis, unbearable relationship or loss does fit into their life. Does it relate to certain themes or patterns of their life? Out of such explorations, clarity and understanding may arise, new orientations or different attitudes develop with which to tackle the next day. Being stopped in one's tracks by illness or life events provides a chance to look at life anew, discover hidden strengths and potential to find new paths to accept and shape one's destiny (Figure 10.1). But equally it is a joint search to find resources and strength to endure suffering and find a deeper relationship to oneself and the world around one in these testing circumstances.

Lievegoed[6,7] explains Steiner's description of the development of the human being in life phases of roughly seven-year periods, each phase having particular

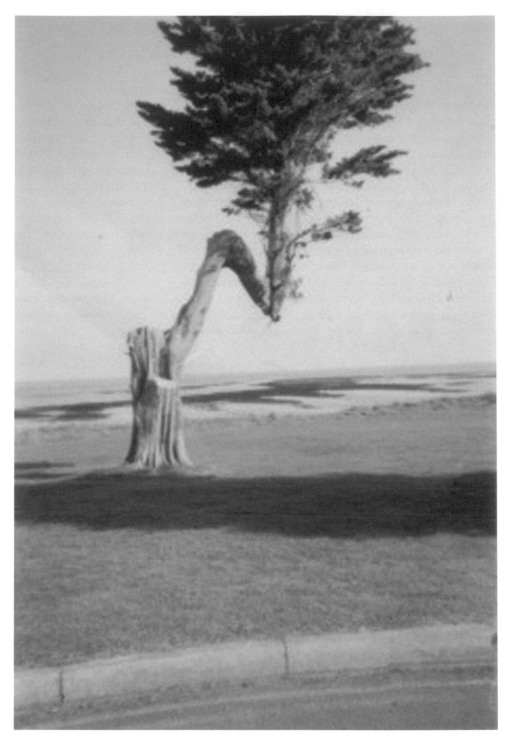

Figure 10.1 *Tree of Life* (John Hazelwood). *See* www.radcliffe-oxford.com/spirituality to view this picture in colour.

tasks that challenge and enrich different parts of our being. Each period is followed by a transition time, which, apart from including the obstacles, joys and challenges that life presents, creates growing points. Insights in life phases provide a backdrop for the biographical counsellor to understand and help the client with the difficulties and challenges on their path.

Another aspect is working with the theme of acceptance and forgiveness. The different religious, spiritual framework or values of patients are taken into account as an essential part of their life. The therapist tries to help patients develop a new relationship with themselves and their world within the context of their belief or value system. When clients lose their way in the maze of life, hit by adversity or lack of health, revealed in illness or depression, they require more than medication to be healed. Illness is a disturbance in the balance between body, soul and spirit, and provides an opportunity to stop, take stock and develop different capabilities. Health and prosperity may make us happy, but pain and suffering connect us deeply with that which is truly human. It can open our inner eyes to see depth and beauty and help us grow inner wings.

Reference has already been made to the three different aspects of the soul – *thinking, feeling* and *willing*. The balance between these three qualities differs in each human being and one or the other is often more dominant. They can be compared to three horses that need to be given reign and direction by the charioteer, the ego, that part in us that takes charge of the situation. When observing the difficulties of a client, it can be of great help to see which of the three horses needs strengthening or quieting down.

Biographical counselling can be of great help, but often needs to be accompanied by medicaments for the nervous, rhythmic or metabolic systems. Often the physical and vital life forces of the patient need to be built up first through massage and eurythmy. This can be followed by artistic therapies such as painting, sculpture or music in order to enliven qualities of soul. Counselling can then address the client through consciousness in soul and spirit matters. During that journey the therapist walks together with the patient to help them deal with pain and suffering and hopefully turn these into strength, new sources of inspiration and insights for the future.

Different types of group work
The confidence-building group

One group that ran for 10 years consisted of patients who mainly suffered from phobias, anxieties and depression, and needed to concentrate on building confidence and self-esteem. Weekly meetings combined conversations or outings with an hour of singing. Activity structured in this way is based on the principle of 'breathing in' and 'breathing out'. Conversations, which reflect 'inward-looking' activity, are alternated with 'outward-directed' activities such as outings and trips accessing nature, or tackling particular phobias through shopping, swimming or cultural expeditions. Similarly, there is a rhythm within each weekly session between 'talking', observation exercises and 'artistic' activity such as singing.

Group for those with cancer

In 2000, a new initiative – Oasis Cancer Support – was set up for groups of people affected by cancer. The aim of this group is to provide a place, like an 'oasis' in the desert, a space in the week where patients can stop at the well, share life stories and fill themselves anew with fresh water, friendship, new insights and inspiration while on their challenging cancer journey. All groups at Blackthorn are structured. The Oasis weekly, two-hour meetings consist of three components:

- social sharing and support
- biographical conversations
- artistic activities.

Participants take part for a year in a group facilitated by one or more therapists. They then 'graduate' into the next phase. This means that a number of the group turn their attention to other activities in their life or can choose to continue together under their own steam. The groups also become smaller in size due to deteriorating health or death of members. Group work is beneficial to patients either in addition to individual treatment or as a separate type of therapy. Support and care for each other and the development of friendships that extend outside the group meetings can become vital ingredients in people's lives.

However, the 'biographical' conversations are equally important. These conversations are not so much about cancer, but touch on aspects of patients' lives, such as their habits, events and values, trust, confidence, celebrations, key decisions and meetings. For patients, sharing their story and listening to the way six or seven other people have dealt with similar situations provides powerful insights and new initiatives when shared with this 'second family' – as patients often call these Oasis groups. Group work creates quite astonishing possibilities for acceptance and change.

Lastly, the exposure of people to artistic work, be it poetry, work with pastels, paint and clay, or improvising with musical instruments, is beneficial. Artistic work not only quietens the interesting and moving conversations, it also creates an opportunity to 'breathe out'. Quietness allows the rediscovery of the immensely healing and nourishing power of the creative forces that live (mostly slumbering) within us.

Cancer has a major impact on people's lives and makes them aware of what is essential and inessential. This new consciousness can have a healing effect. Sharing these discoveries in group work and being part of the community can be of major benefit for all those involved, patients, carers and health professionals alike.

Issues of fear and hope are important topics in this work. Hope is not necessarily a concept concerned with getting better or having a quantity of time. When suffering and death are not pushed out as unwanted enemies or subjects of taboo, then hope and life can take on different colours and meaning. In the Oasis groups there is space and time to share fears and struggles, or there may be discussion about what might follow after death. Listening to other patients' 'hopes' and views, be it acceptance, fighting, humour or great inspirations, often liberates people from their isolation and fears, widening their horizons. Hope and meaning can shape and influence the quality of *each day* of an individual life and the relationship that individual shares with others *now*. This is true regardless of whether an individual has two weeks or many years to live. Hope has to do with owning fully what life presents and becoming creative with it. Often patients will say: 'I certainly did not want the cancer, but I would not have missed this year; so much has happened, I have experienced so much love, I have made new friends; life has become worthwhile, whereas before I took everything for granted. Now I know again what is essential and what is totally trivial.'

Rudolf Steiner[8] describes the need to develop an attitude of gratitude for whatever life has brought, for all positive things as well as for the great difficulties and challenges. Further, he advocates the need to develop the will to connect strongly with events in the present, in the here and now. In doing so, an individual's capabilities and faculties will be forged in their soul and provide confidence, trust and the ability to meet whatever challenge may come.

Other forms of group work

In most therapies the emphasis is on one-to-one work, exploring and accompanying the individual patient on their unique journey. The Blackthorn team has developed group work for counselling, art and music therapy as a response to growing pressure to make space for new patients needing individual therapy. A number of patients need a longer period of therapy, but not necessarily on a one-to-one basis.

Small art classes gave rise to art history groups and have resulted in art excursions. These have included trips to London and abroad; to the cathedral of Chartres, and the art treasures in Florence and Greece. The healing aspect of looking at truly great art was already well discovered in the Middle Ages, when patients were brought in front of the Isenheimer Altar in Colmar in France. Exposing patients to works of art gives the soul a chance to expand and be touched by the dimensions of divine inspiration and imagination. These excursions also bring healing through the joys and challenges of travelling together, but also in patients finding dimensions of beauty and wonder within themselves hitherto not experienced.

Music groups have proven to be beneficial in a number of ways. Making music without having to know a specific instrument or use written sheet music is a great revelation. Patients develop a new ear for rhythm and a sense of time, which is so deeply disturbed by the stress and pace of contemporary life and results in a host of illnesses in the soul's rhythmic system. Individuals working with percussion instruments or playing with simple hand lyres learn about themselves and learn to listen to each other. Some groups have performed in care homes for the elderly or in hospices. These performances have resulted in confidence building and greater self-worth through being of service to others. The group provides a structured setting in which these discoveries are made.

Eurythmy is a specific form of movement, which has been derived from the universal origins of speech and music. The therapy employs music, speech and poetry to facilitate the teaching of its exercises and lays particular emphasis on the rhythm, balance and harmony of the movement. Daily practice is required for the patient to begin to feel more 'at one' with themselves and their body. This can be experienced in improved posture, co-ordination and gait. The way a person takes hold of their body in movement reflects who they are and how they feel. Most of the curative work happens in one-to-one treatment in precise movements and exercises indicated for specific physical conditions. However, eurythmy in small groups is also employed for performances at festivals throughout the year. These demand a great presence of mind and awareness in performing movements together with others.

Conclusion

In this chapter I have tried to show how conventional medicine in a NHS practice can be extended by the use of anthroposophical therapies and medical interventions by a team of doctors and therapists testing and researching the philosophical ideas of Rudolf Steiner. In this approach, spirituality is to do with a faithful determination, an attitude that wishes to explore how man exists as a microcosm of the macrocosm that is the universe.

Steiner indicates that with the development of consciousness the task for the twenty-first century is to integrate religion, science and the arts in a new way. Spirituality is not a veneer of a mundane daily existence. Nor is spirituality something different on Sunday or Monday depending on what activity is undertaken. 'Spirit is never without matter and matter never without spirit.' Daily grey routine can be enlivened and lit up with inner substance and new insights. The inner sun of our being, when nurtured and exercised, can shine when the outer glorious sun is behind the clouds. The integration of religion, science and art can become a matter of inspiration and imagination, combining the visible and invisible realties of life, which when penetrated by conscious effort, bring healing and wellbeing in the development of humanity. In the work at Blackthorn Medical Centre, the main emphasis is on addressing the uniqueness of each individual on their journey to further development and 'being well', whether this takes place in consultations with the doctor, in the one-to-one therapy sessions, group work or in rehabilitation work in Blackthorn's garden.

The challenge of illness and adversity creates the chance to find a new balance between body, soul and spirit. Doctors and therapists stand by with expertise, love and time to offer guidance to patients who wish to influence their life and destiny through their own activity and take steps towards the unfolding of their own true being.

References

1   Steiner R (1994) *Theosophy.* Anthroposophic Press, Gt Barrington, Massachusetts.
2   www.eurythmy.org.uk
3   Douch G (2004) *Medicine for the Whole Person, A Guide to Anthroposophical Treatment.* Floris Books, Edinburgh.
4   McGavin D (2001) *Primary Care Cancer Pilot.* Unpublished, Blackthorn Trust.
5   Evans M, Rodger I (1992) *Anthroposophical Medicine, Healing for Body, Soul and Spirit.* Thoresens, London.
6   Lievegoed B (1997) *Phases.* Rudolf Steiner Press, London.
7   Lievegoed B (1985) *Man on the Threshold.* Hawthorn Press, Stroud.
8   Steiner R (1989) *Early Death and Cosmic Life: lecture Berlin 19th March 1918.* Spiritual Research Editions, New York, NY.

Sources of further information

Adult education
Website: www.emerson.org.uk

Anthroposophical medicine
The Anthroposophical Medical Association
Park Attwood Clinic
Trimpley, Bewdley, Worcs DY12 1RE
Tel: 01299 861444
Email: movementoffice@btinternet.com

Architecture
Section for the Visual Arts
C/o Camphill Architects Newton Dee Bielside
Aberdeen AB15 9DX
Tel: 01244 867450
Email: wolo.r@virgin.net

Arts
Painting and sculpture
Tobias School of Art
Coombe Hill Rd
East Grinstead, W Sussex RH19 4LZ
Tel/fax: 01342 313655

Hibernia School of Artistic Therapy
Centre for Science and Art, Lansdown
Stroud, Glos GL5 1BB
Tel: 01453 751685
Website: www.anth.org.uk/hibernia

Biodynamic agriculture
The Biodynamic Agricultural Association
Painswick Inn Project, Gloucester Street
Stroud, Glos GL5 1QG
Tel/fax: 01453 759501
Email: bdaa@biodynamic.freeserve.co.uk
Website: www.anth.org.uk/biodynamic

Blackthorn Trust
Blackthorn Medical Centre
St Andrews Road
Maidstone, Kent ME16 9AN
Website: www.blackthorn.org.uk

Biographical counselling
Biography and Social Development Trust
First North Hillside House, Lewes Road
Forest Row, Sussex RH18 5ES
Tel: 01342 822907
Website: www.biographywork.org
Email: biogsoctru@aol.com

Eurythmy
Website: www.eurythmy.org.uk

Medicines and bodycare
Weleda (UK) Ltd
Ilkeston, Derbyshire DE7 8DR
Tel: 0115 944 8200
Fax: 0115 944 8210
Email: WeledaUK@compuserve.com
Website: www.weleda.co.uk

Special needs
The Association of Camphill Communities
Garwain House, 56 Welham Road
Norton Malton, N Yorks YO17 9PD
Email: info@camphill.org.uk

Waldorf education
Steiner Waldorf Fellowship
Kidbrooke Park
Forest Row, Sussex RH18 5JB
Tel: 01342 822115
Email: mail@waldorf.compulink.co.uk
Website: www.steinerwaldorf.org.uk

CHAPTER 11

Art as therapy

Hazel Adams

Introduction

This chapter begins by considering the role of art in relation to spirituality from a historical perspective that reflects a shift from art as an integral part of life to the contemporary view of art as anything original. Art therapy using an anthroposophical approach is then considered and exemplified using illustrative case studies. Because of the difficulties of reproducing the nuances of colour in patient's art work in text the paintings can be viewed on the web at www.radcliffe-oxford.com/spirituality. Therefore this chapter is best read alongside a computer that gives access to this website.

Development of consciousness

In ancient cultures, art was an integral part of life, which permeated and informed all levels of society.[1] Art, science and religion were a unity and the idea that these different aspects could be seen separately had not yet arisen. In ancient Egypt, the Pharaoh was regarded as a god, and was still attuned to the spiritual world in a direct way. The priests conducted the science of medicine and practised temple healings that involved inducing a deep sleep during which the priest was able to bring about organic changes. They also held a vast knowledge of poisonous substances and their therapeutic application. All the practical decisions regarding external life were guided from the priest/king domain.

In contrast, during the Greek epoch, a transition in consciousness gradually unfolds, moving from the portrayal of emotions as external figures on the stage in Greek mystery dramas to the emergence of philosophical questioning. Hence actors wore masks depicting particular emotions on the stage, such as the furies (anger), illustrating externally what later became experienced and owned by the individual. During this time the healing methods no longer involved a temple sleep, but still embodied a holistic approach. Mystery centres were sources of spiritual knowledge where initiation rituals were practised and informed the social and cultural life at the time. The temple at Epidaurus was such a mystery centre where healing took place and involved the patient in a wide range of treatment. Dream-states revealed to the healer the necessary plants for remedies. Also, attending performances of mystery dramas enabled a cathartic process to facilitate healing.

In Greek culture, from about the fourth century BC, the unfolding of individual thinking and philosophical debate gradually emerged. Great philosophers forged a path that resulted in a shift from the divine, kingly inspired consciousness, with which people complied with a childlike obedience, to a sound and thorough examination of thinking. This resulted in mankind losing touch with the divine. Rather than the Egyptian view reflected in the hymns in the *Book of the Dead*, which demonstrated a certainty and far greater value on the life to come, the Greek view became that of Homer: 'better a beggar on earth, than a king in the realm of shades'. However, the idea that knowledge discovered in the mystery centres could simply be made available to all people still did not exist and betrayal of the mysteries was a crime punishable by death. Socrates was found guilty of this crime and sentenced to death by poisoning, as described in Plato's *Phaedo*.[2]

Art was considered an essential element connecting the spiritual world and earthly life, and demonstrates the differing levels of consciousness that existed in various historic epochs. For example, in the most primitive sculpture, human form is conveyed as a fecund goddess figure, archetype of fertility, life and its renewal. In contrast, Egyptian figures are formal and of huge dimensions (e.g. sphinx), stylistic, depicting a king as a deity with a forward-looking gaze reaching far into the future, yet encompassing the past. The Greek era saw a change in size of sculptures towards more human proportions with flowing garments and asymmetry strongly represented. The sculptures of human figures were personifications of the elements or of the Gods, showing a harmony and balance unsurpassed and reappearing in post-Christian art of the high renaissance, for example, in the work of Michaelangelo.

For the Greeks, beauty was essential to health, an ingredient without which one could not find humanity. Sculptures tend to depict the ideal or spiritual archetype, whereas by Roman times they come under the direct influence of personality, with lifelike portrayals of individuals. However, the post-Christian art found in the catacombs in Rome conveys a new simplistic style, demonstrating an almost child-like naivety. The heights of technical ability achieved hitherto have vanished, but gradually emerge again in a profound expression of spirituality in the early icon paintings. The practice of treating the background of these paintings with gold leaf can be seen as a manifestation of another level of consciousness, gold expressing directly the awareness of the divine world out of which the Icon emanates, whereas a blue background depicting the sky, reflecting a more earthly consciousness, generally only begins to appear in works of the thirteenth century.

Until the 1600s, painting largely, but not exclusively, depicts spiritual events. For many years paintings were the main source of portraying the content of the life of Christ and his disciples and the reality of spiritual hierarchies. These guided the whole populace to an understanding of the spiritual world through the picture, as access to the written word was available only to specific groups within society. Gradually human beings became even more separate from their spiritual identity. Art, science and religion emerged as clearly demarcated areas of life. This division of consciousness was an inevitable consequence of an increasing awareness of earthly laws. This is evidenced in all the scientific discoveries now taken for granted, for example the laws of gravity, relativity, electricity, steam power and all that has followed since.

These new insights were accompanied by a reduction of direct spiritual perception. Indeed, the principles laid down by Francis Bacon[3] made it impossible to be certain about anything that could not be weighed or measured. The consequence of this approach has led to a contemporary consciousness that demands a questioning philosophy. So, mankind has moved from direct perception of the Gods, to belief in a spiritual world, and finally to denial of all that cannot be proved by earthly laws or perceptions. This historic process has played a vital role in humans developing independent judgement, and thereby a path towards true freedom. Freedom in this context is not intended to imply acting in selfish isolation, but in harmony with others and the earth itself, as described by Rudolf Steiner in his major philosophical work, *The Philosophy of Freedom*.[4] This new path to higher consciousness, however, is not automatic, but one needing recognition and individual will.

Contemporary secular society

Currently, the momentum of scientific and technological achievements has resulted in choices that are both beneficial and demanding. These advances enable human beings to access a broad spectrum of life options but also involve huge responsibilities and ethical questions. Scientific discovery tends to take precedence over many other aspects of life. Although some scientists encompass both artistic flair and imagination, or a mood of spirituality in their work, generally, science exists as a separate discipline and is not obliged to consider either artistic or spiritual perspectives. This is exemplified in the rigour of quantitative studies that provide empirical evidence-based data, such as that found in the double-blind trial, as being the most highly esteemed research method. The idea of the inclusion of self in research requires a spiritual view of the human being to make real sense. Since we have largely eliminated this aspect in science the human being is excluded. Qualitative research that seeks to redress this imbalance has been conducted into anthroposophic medicine.[5] There are also occasions when medical or scientific experts and artists chose to work together or are embodied in the same person. One example can be seen in the courtyard of the Royal Brompton Hospital, London, which houses a sculpture using a water flow-form to express in an artistic medium the powerful dynamics of the heart. The artist, Philip Kilner, is also a research scientist.

While modern science demands strict lawfulness (i.e. evidence-based outcomes), art on the other hand has developed a tendency to flout laws, some modern artists creating individual modes of expression with the commonly held view that anything original is art. Consequently, the role of beauty and associated aesthetic considerations tend to be repressed or considered outmoded. The psychologist James Hillman describes this in his essay 'The Practice of Beauty',[6] in which he postulates that love can only be present at the hand of beauty; beauty itself defies definition in mere words but is a deep inner human experience. As art portrays the changing consciousness of historical epochs, contemporary work reflects a high degree of individualisation. Art has in some instances become divorced from its spiritual origins, as is evident in the use of art merely to make political statements or promote consumerism. However, the understanding that works of art may reveal spiritual inspiration is growing, and individuals are fascinated by the creative and spiritual experiences of the modern artist. The closer the artist comes to a true expression of a spiritual law expressed through his free creativity, the greater the possibility for others to unite with it, because these laws form the basis of all creation. In other words, the respect and understanding of the laws of colour or geometrical composition do not inhibit creativity or push it into a false aestheticism, but rather set the artist free to create, just as knowledge of musical laws enables a composer to be highly inventive. The following illustrates this well:

> Art enables us to find ourselves and lose ourselves at the same time. The mind that responds to the intellectual and spiritual values that lie hidden in a poem, a painting, or a piece of music, discovers a spiritual vitality that lifts it above itself, takes it out of itself, and makes it present to itself on a level of being that it did not know it could ever achieve.[7] (p.29)

Currently, the growing idea that human deeds and creations have a global impact is conveyed in an increased awareness of ecological concerns and the collective responsibility of humanity for the preservation and respect for the earth as a living organism. Many new art forms reflect these contemporary concerns, for example nature sculptures and installation art using organic materials such as driftwood, stones, leaves and ice. Similarly, landscape sculptures[8,9] reflect these values. An example is Udo Zembok's planned Glass Sun-observatory in Brugge, Belgium (Figure 11.1), designed to cast a coloured, elongated shadow over the earth and be particularly striking at the winter solstice.

Many traditional forms of religious devotion and worship are falling away, with significant numbers of people having no religion or basic education in religious history. The current age, defined by Rudolf Steiner as the 'consciousness soul',[10] demands awareness and testing of ideas as opposed to compliantly believing them. Therefore many religious doctrines are being challenged by this changing consciousness. On the one hand man is freer than before and yet also locked into systems, which are largely material and economically driven, that impose strong limitations on the development of free creativity. For instance, the economic demands on an individual are often experienced as placing severe restrictions on how they may express their contribution to working life from a spiritual perspective. Attempts to remedy this are evidenced in the growing number of people seeking to change their lifestyle, relocating in order to come closer to their true values. There seems to be an increasing interest in the spiritual dimension, with explorations into many different forms of spiritual practice, which reflects a search or longing for a dimension outside the material.

Using art in therapy

Experience in therapeutic work over several years has shown that illnesses and life crises potentially lead to a quest for meaning. At times of great testing, consciousness is jolted, shifted from the mundane and routine into an existential search. A review of life's achievements and shortcomings may lead to a new or heightened awareness of spirituality. This may also happen at times of joyful events, such as the birth of a child or the meeting of a person with whom we form a close connection. Similarly, awareness of the spiritual may come from a series of events where the synchronicity is breathtaking. These are often passed off as coincidences, but it is difficult to discount the working of a higher wisdom. For example, a woman who made a point of never missing a train, on one occasion, following numerous incidents that were apparent hindrances, missed her train by just a few minutes. The train crashed, with many losing their lives.

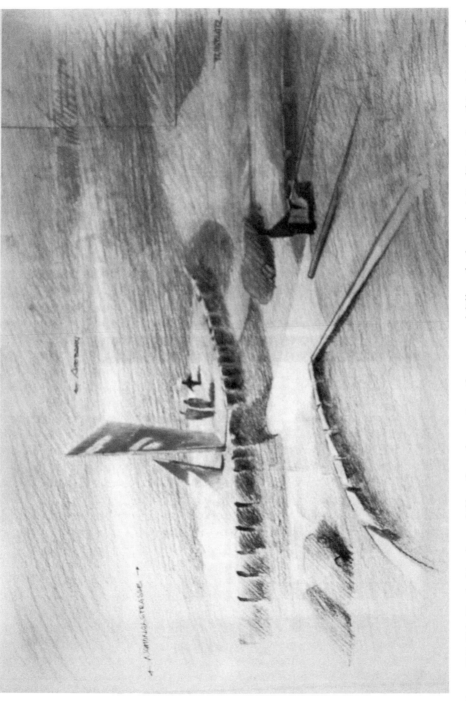

Figure 11.1 Udo Zembok's planned Glass Sun-observatory. *See* www.radcliffe-oxford.com/spirituality to view this picture in colour.

Our perceptions of life events are not compelled, but determined by choice and our awareness of the wider spiritual perspective of life. Each individual human being is unfolding at their own pace and from where they are standing on their life's journey they may either see an event negatively, for example that an illness is simply unfair, or as bad luck or positively, as an opportunity to bring change, to take stock, to find or develop new capabilities. When confronted by severe difficulties, an individual's world is turned upside down, values are examined afresh, what seemed important suddenly appears insignificant. In these circumstances some may find themselves in need of help to manage anger, blame, guilt or depression to name but a few of the wide range of emotional responses possible.

Similarly, our response to art is not compelled, and it is also able to evoke moods we find surprising, emotions we did not expect. When we encounter a work of art we can pass it by or become interested for as long or short a time as we choose. The work will convey only as much as we are able to perceive at that point of our development. Completely new aspects are often experienced in a later encounter with the same work. This is because new levels of awareness arise over time, as we ourselves are changing constantly, even when we are not aware of it. We may, for example, look at a painting and see only its physical properties, but in later observation be deeply struck by the expression in the eyes, the gesture of the hands or how one figure relates to another, which is influenced by our own experiences in the intervening period. This enables art to be a highly flexible tool in a therapeutic process in which perceptions are gradually awakened, allowing engagement with the work at varying levels of intensity appropriate to the individual's current state of consciousness. There is no compulsion in the artistic therapy process, but with gentle support and appropriate guidance, the patient or client's artwork uncovers the mystery of their problems. This is dependent on client/patient levels of perception and their consequent awareness of what is revealed.

The therapist's experience helps to identify where the client is in the process of using art as therapy and enable them to take new steps. For example, a client may present blaming their current difficulties on another person. During the therapeutic process they may become aware of their own role in the situation, moving from the position of victim to one of taking responsibility for their own responses. This may arise through their experience of approaching an artistic problem. If this does not resolve in the way they would like it to, the therapist may help them to gradually become aware of their own potential through moving the artwork forward by identifying self-imposed obstacles to progress.

Anthroposophical approach

The anthroposophical approach to art therapy enhances the spiritual and soul aspect of the human being. There are many modalities within art therapy, with a wide range of application supported by different theoretical models. Broadly presented, there is the psychodynamic approach (Freudian), analytic therapy (Jungian), the humanistic, which includes Rogers' person-centred expressive arts therapy, psycho-educational, systemic and integrative approaches.[11] In an anthroposophical approach, the individual's spiritual foundation is central to art therapy. Whereas many approaches to art therapy work with the psychological aspects of the individual as separate from their physical body, the anthroposophical approach takes note of the relationship of the physical and life (physiological) processes with those of the soul and spirit.[12]

The soul embodies feelings and emotions furnishing the ego with experiences. The ego, representing the spiritual aspect of the individual, is eternal. The basic premise is that physical illnesses have their seat in the activity of the soul, either in this lifetime, for example shock resulting in palpitations, or of the soul disposition as it has lived in previous incarnations, for example a life-threatening illness.[13] However, traditionally classified mental illnesses have their basis in subtle dysfunctions of one or other of the main bodily organs, for example some forms of depression may be related to liver function. The role of the art therapist is to contribute to sharing with the physician and other colleagues thoughts on where the seat of activity that has resulted in the ill health of their client/patient lies, where the disharmony in the interplay between body and soul arises. This determines the choice of artwork that would most benefit the individual. The decision takes into account resources available and agreement of the client/patient. The aims of treatment have to be clear, but the means of achievement are always open to negotiation and discovery.

Historically, the myths and legends of many cultures express how colour intimately reflects the soul life of the human being. In Norse mythology, the rainbow is the bridge between the physically manifest world and the Gods, it provides access between the two. In the Bible, it is God's covenant with man after the great flood. In von Goethe's fairy tale 'The Green Snake & the Beautiful Lily',[14] it becomes a bridge which man is able to cross and regain access to the spiritual world. Colour is therefore not representative or symbolic, but *is* the soul life of the world and of man himself. The objective of therapy is to help the individual gain greater self-awareness through enlivening their soul/spiritual dimension, which is always present, but is asleep, dreaming or deeply blocked for various reasons. Finding a pathway to deeper layers of consciousness can lead ultimately to an awakening of the true individuality. Awareness of spiritual reality may open up readily if the environment is suitably nurturing. Inklings of this deeper consciousness exist in everyone and are illustrated in poetry of the romantic period, such as that of William Wordsworth's 'Ode to Immortality'.

> Our birth is but a sleep and a forgetting;
> the Soul that rises with us, our life's Star,
> hath had elsewhere its setting,
> and cometh from afar;
> Not in entire forgetfulness,
> And not in utter nakedness,
> But trailing clouds of Glory do we come
> From God, who is our home.[15]

However, speaking of spiritual matters directly may evoke sceptical responses in present-day culture. Patients report feelings of isolation if these newly acquired levels of self-discovery are discredited or scorned by those closest to them. The experience of illness impacts on all those involved with the patient, and their new perceptions may be provocative for others, causing discomfort, which may result in the need for further support. During the art therapy process it is noteworthy how often patients tentatively mention something of a spiritual experience, maybe quite small, which they have never dared to share for fear of being regarded as mentally unsound or suddenly religious. That such innocent experiences have to be kept from others is now changing, but still depends on the individual situation, and adds to the challenges encountered in the journey through an illness. These experiences include encountering spiritual or angelic beings, experiencing the presence of one departed who is offering help or protection in times of danger, or waking visions of past historical periods in which scenes arise involving the individual in an entirely different mode of existence. They may also include simply feeling oneself on a different level of inner experience. The depth of relief expressed by patients reveals a fundamental human need to share experiences with one who is able to remain open to these revelations without judging or negating them. The practice of art itself helps to build a bridge of understanding, of empathy, because creativity defies categorising experiences narrowly. This arises naturally during an art session that begins with a specific theme and colours, but the creation itself only emerges as the work progresses. This is because art cannot be 'thought out', but arises and is perceived in the creative act.

The nourishment that comes to the soul through working with colour, discovering its nature and laws, creating in the moment and transforming the ugly and disappointing aspects of the work into something expressing beauty, cannot be underestimated. The work of James Hillman[16] proves helpful in this respect. He proposes that in contemporary culture beauty is repressed, and that without beauty love cannot unfold. Without love we cannot care properly for the physical world, ourselves or others, or find a living connection to the spiritual world. There are aspects in his work that concur with Steiner's philosophy that in a contemporary, predominantly materialistic culture, everything would depend on whether human beings could develop a new relationship to spiritual life and the world of nature. This demands a shift from a focus purely on rational brain-bound thought, to enabling the heart to develop as an organ of spiritual perception.[17] Through the practice of art therapy the human heart can begin to unfold this perception, not through the avoidance of the ugly, but through the truly spiritual activity of transformation; owning what is ugly and working on its transformation potentially leads to beneficial metamorphosis.

Case studies

The two cases outlined below describe examples of the process of change effected by art therapy. They illustrate quite different modes of expression. They have been selected to demonstrate how art therapy can be beneficial to patients with vastly different levels of spiritual challenge.

Jean

Jean, aged 52 years, was happily married and had no children. Diagnosed with breast cancer some time ago, she had received all the necessary treatments, but now had metastases. She was small and frail in appearance with a beautiful, open, childlike smile, and gently spoken, expressing dismay at finding herself in this situation. She had been a librarian for many years and although not enthusiastic about the job had enjoyed the social rapport with colleagues. From her perspective life had been fairly happy and relatively uncomplicated. She wanted to improve what was sometimes a difficult and painful relationship with a sibling. She did not regret being childless and was very happy with her partner and he with her. Illness had intruded like a sudden dark cloud into an otherwise comfortable life. She struggled to make sense of it and come to terms with the fact that her lifespan would be shorter than she had anticipated. She was not so much afraid of death as the process of dying and her ability to endure pain. She was an agnostic and so the spiritual dimension of life was open for exploration. She was impressed by the way a young colleague had managed her journey through illness to death and had come seeking the same help for her own situation.

Jean immediately took to painting and revealed a love of colour, but had no expectation of any artistic ability. Confessing to being a bit of a 'shopaholic', she described shopping as satisfying her need to see and touch different colours and textures, without necessarily buying.

Beginning with the technique of wet on wet, which helps the colours spread easily and avoids feelings of uncertainty about what shapes or forms might arise, she readily took up the brush. She demonstrated an ability to blend her colours well, even at the first session, although she applied them thinly and the painting had a 'washed-out' appearance that reflected her physical weakness and low energy (Figure 11.2 Early painting – *see* www.radcliffe-oxford.com/spirituality). In the first sessions she was happy to paint simple colour washes. Working with the mood of morning, the atmosphere she created was calm and thoughtful. Tiredness sometimes made progress very slow, but she was not impatient and did not become frustrated.

With growing confidence came a wish to paint a tree landscape (Figure 11.3 Tree landscape – *see* www.radcliffe-oxford.com/spirituality). Jean needed some assistance, but she was pleased with the result. Gradually her physical strength improved and she began to smile and enjoy her sessions, expressing a naive delight and surprise at her hitherto undiscovered creativity.

The flower pictures, inspired by various posies on the art room table, were entirely her choice of subject. The painting of apricot roses was a high point (Figure 11.4 Apricot rose – *see* www.radcliffe-oxford.com/spirituality). She had learned to form the leaves and flowers from varying colour shades, making forms become visible by painting planes of colour rather than a solid outline. This unlocked a childlike wonder and an increased awareness of the colours surrounding her in nature. She became aware that previously she had stared at her surroundings rather than looking at them consciously; now she was able to see colour variations in the sky and their seasonal changes.

On completion of the first rose picture a new step was taken to soften the form and enter more deeply into uniting with the flower rather than looking at it (Figure 11.5 Fading rose into colour – *see* www.radcliffe-oxford.com/spirituality). This was a difficult and significant step for Jean because adults tend to 'look at' the world as observers rather than uniting with it.

The next series of paintings are remarkable for their intensity of colour, mood and quality of blending. Jean worked diligently to gain mastery in this work and had great satisfaction with the results (Figure 11.6 Autumn – *see* www.radcliffe-oxford.com/spirituality).

In her painting to create a Christmas mood (Figure 11.7 Christmas mood – *see* www.radcliffe-oxford.com/spirituality), she worked at the weaving of light and warmth into darkness, which she found most satisfying. Her painting explored the mood of Christmas as a festival, giving the possibility of a rebirth of inner light and warmth. She was not embarrassed to explore such possibilities in the privacy of the therapy session. Any resistance was directed towards more traditional religious forms of expression of spirituality because this might alienate her from others.

Weaving light and warmth together in a harmonious way is often very difficult to achieve, especially in the case of cancer, where there is a tendency to paint the light and warmth with a heavy or physical quality. The warmth may become stone-like and separated off from the light, instead of gently suffusing the whole picture. Jean's latter paintings were inspired by a beautiful coloured shell from South Africa, which was lying on the table. On picking it up she described her love of these colours and how she wished to find and paint them. Jean managed to do this really well (Figure 11.8 Final three paintings based on shell – *see* www.radcliffe-oxford.com/spirituality). By this time she was seriously ill, and her artistic sensitivity and achievements increased as her physical condition deteriorated. Her spirituality became more available and present, although not at a fully conscious level, through the qualitative mood she exuded. Towards the end of her life her physical body was so frail she was unable to open the door without help, but she determinedly attended her sessions every week until shortly before her death, which came with relative peace.

During the therapy sessions she spoke of smoothing the problems with her close relative, and although tearful at first, became increasingly free to view the problem from different angles, with more freedom and understanding of the need for considered response rather than immediate reaction.

The aims in this particular case were as follows:

- to create an awareness and development of her true potential (which accelerated closer to her death)
- to enhance her sense of self and her ability to find the challenges and work with these in a positive mood
- to experience her individuality as having meaning, and to contemplate the possibility of a future consciousness free of the physical body.

In experiencing a divine spark within oneself, it becomes possible to develop a relationship to the divine and spiritual world. Jean left this world unfolding and exploring. Jean demonstrated that in working with the medium of colour she was able to take steps in building a bridge from sensory experience to the spiritual world of her future existence.

Beth

Beth was in her early thirties and presented suffering panic attacks, extreme exhaustion and complete collapse. She had lost confidence, was very pale, with a drained and empty expression, and gave the impression of suffering from a deep tiredness. Her smile was thin and delicate, as if it was an effort. She had been a hardworking, conscientious person and suddenly, after a rather uneventful illness, could not recover. The diagnosis was myalgic encephalopathy (ME). Her working life was intellectually oriented, not particularly balanced by art, music or other relaxing hobbies. Work, housework and social events that she felt obliged to fulfil dominated her life. She had become fearful of going abroad for holidays in case she had panic attacks, and found this very limiting.

Interestingly, her first paintings (Figure 11.9 First two paintings – *see* www. radcliffe-oxford.com/spirituality) showed a lot of activity, not reflecting tiredness, but very active, yet not integrated, reminiscent of unco-ordinated energy. This conveyed a picture of excessive metabolic activity with no space for rest, and was in complete contrast to her actual appearance.

Gradually, she worked from wet painting to a dry medium, using pastel to gain more mastery and a less nebulous quality in her work (Figure 11.10 Pastels – *see* www.radcliffe-oxford.com/spirituality). The more focused she became, the less panicky she felt. Her panic attacks could be regarded as excessive, undirected, unconscious energy. Her unused imaginative capacities had begun to appear organically (in panic attacks) and needed to be harnessed in a creative format. The therapy was to assist in directing these forces and focusing them, but at the same time give the nurturing support of colour rather than drawing or charcoal.

Gradually she gained the strength to take control of her life again (Figure 11.11 Copy of work by August Macke – *see* www.radcliffe-oxford.com/spirituality), but saw the need to understand herself better in order to be effective in life. Until this event she had moved through life without much consciousness of herself or any deeper issues.

Questions of spiritual development now came to the fore and she worked on some of the basic exercises given by Steiner for overcoming nervousness.[18] She now saw herself as a key player in the way forward, rather than a sufferer. Her next step in therapeutic work was in music therapy, and this proved extremely helpful to her. Spiritual development in its broadest sense involves unfolding awareness. There are no limits to how far this may go, but it cannot be forced without negative results. The arts do not force or coerce, but gently guide the individual's inner experience towards a closer connection with its origins, at their chosen pace. The therapist is a facilitator for this process and respects each person's need to unfold at a different rate and in varying degrees. Although therapy is prescribed for particular illnesses, the therapist adapts the nature of delivery, which is determined by the individuality of each patient. Although there are definite general tendencies accompanying an illness, the way through these tendencies has to be found anew for each person. One works towards renewed health by fully embracing the current situation as the starting point.

Conclusion

The artistic practice required by the therapist is to sensitively assess the needs presented by the patient, to hear their aims and longings and help them translate these into creative activity that may work into the organic life of the body. The therapeutic process is as much a challenge for the therapist as the patient, and requires them to continue personal and professional development in order to sustain their work. The practice of meditation, study and one's own artistic discoveries are a necessary part of this development. The therapist's privilege is to accompany the patient and share the sense of achievement as the artistic process unfolds new insights and initiatives that had once seemed unattainable.

References

1 Richter G (1982) *Art and Human Consciousness*. Anthroposophic Press, New York, NY.
2 Livingstone RW (1944) *Life of Socrates – Plato – Phaedo*. Clarendon Press, Oxford.
3 Bacon F (1620) *Novum Organum*. Open Court Pub (1994), Chicago, Illinois.
4 Steiner R (1964) *The Philosophy of Freedom*. Rudolph Steiner Press, London, Chapter 9.
5 Ritchie J, Wilkinson J, Gantley M *et al.* (2001) *A Model of Integrated Primary Care; Anthroposophic Medicine*. National Centre for Social Research and Queen Mary, University of London.
6 Hillman J (Undated) The Practice of Beauty. *Resurgence*. **157**: 34–7.
7 Merton T (1955) *No Man is an Island*. Hollis and Carter, London.
8 Goldworthy A (1990) *Andy Goldworthy*. Viking, Penguin Books, London.
9 Nash D (1993) *At the Edge of the Forest*. Annely Juda Gina Art catalogue.
10 Lievegoed B (1984) *Man on the Threshold*. Hawthorn Press, Stroud.
11 Rubin JA (2001) *Approaches to Art Therapy*. Brunner-Routledge, London.
12 Steiner R (2000) *The Healing Process*. Anthroposophic Press, New York, NY, Lecture 5.
13 Steiner R (1952) *Man's Life on Earth and in the Spiritual World*. Anthroposophical Publishing, London.
14 von Goethe JW (1979) *The Green Snake & the Beautiful Lily* (1795). Floris Books, Edinburgh.
15 William Wordsworth (1992) *Ode to Immortality*. Aurum Press, London.
16 Hillman J (1982) *The Thought of the Heart and the Soul of the World*. Spring Publications, Woodstock, Connecticut.
17 Cottrell AP (1982) *Goethe's View of Evil*. Floris Books, Edinburgh.
18 Steiner R (1995) *Anthroposophy in Everyday Life*. Anthroposophic Press, New York, NY.

CHAPTER 12

Music and wellbeing

Stephen Clift and Grenville Hancox

Life without music is simply an error, a pain, an exile.

Frederick Nietzsche

Introduction

There is a growing consensus that spirituality and religious beliefs have a crucial significance in our understanding of health, for processes of healthcare and treatment, and more especially in holistic concepts of 'healing' and coping with long-term and terminal illness.[1–3] In addressing the role that music might play in relation to spirituality and healthcare, it is important to explore the links between spirituality and health, and then between spirituality and music. Important conceptual issues will be considered and significant contributions to research will be reviewed in making a case for the place of music in the context of healthcare.

Spirituality and health

First, how are the connections between spirituality and health to be understood? A good starting point for any discussion of health and its spiritual dimensions is still the definition enshrined over 50 years ago in the preamble to the Constitution of the World Health Organization.[4] Health, it states is:

> ...a state of complete physical, mental and social well-being and not merely an absence of disease or infirmity.

Although this definition is not without its difficulties from a scientific point of view, it continues to provide an inspirational vision, which acknowledges the positive, multidimensional, interactive character of health as a whole, embracing not just physical functioning but also the importance of psychological and social wellbeing.

On the basis of this definition, WHO has pursued a significant research programme aimed at understanding and assessing health-related 'quality of life' (the WHOQOL project). In presenting an account of this work, Power *et al.*[5] note:

> ...that quality of life is a patient-perceived multi-dimensional construct that encompasses an evaluation of at least three basic aspects of quality of life: namely emotional well-being, physical state and social functioning. (p.495)

What is most striking about the WHO work, is the fact that the data gathered from around the world:

> ...show that the basic understanding of factors inherent to quality of life does not differ substantially across cultures... (p.504)

Initially, the WHOQOL research identified 'spirituality' as one of six facets of the psychological domain of health, constituting spirituality/religion/personal beliefs. More recently, the project has given closer attention to the significance of spirituality for health, and a new 32-item questionnaire relating specifically to 'spirituality, religiousness and personal beliefs' (WHOQOL-SRPB) has been developed from an extensive pilot test of 105 questions in 18 centres around the world.[6] Spirituality/Religion/Personal Beliefs is now regarded as a separate domain within the WHO model, and is defined by eight facets:

- spiritual connection
- meaning and purpose in life
- experience of awe and wonder
- wholeness and integration
- spiritual strength
- inner peace
- hope and optimism
- faith.

The WHO project provides both a conceptual clarification, based on research evidence, of the key components of 'spirituality', and adds a new cross-culturally validated research instrument to those already available[3] that can be used to research the significance of spiritual and religious beliefs for health and healthcare outcomes.

The importance of spirituality and spiritual issues in the context of healthcare and for wellbeing and recovery of patients is widely recognised. In a recent editorial, Culliford[1] questions the validity of mechanistic medical models and argues for a wider recognition of the role of such factors as 'faith, hope and compassion in the healing process'. He cites the major review undertaken by Koenig *et al.*[7] as providing 'a critical, systematic, and comprehensive analysis of the empirical research, examining relations between religion or spirituality and many physical and mental health conditions', which highlights a consistent pattern of better health among those with religious or spiritual convictions. The value of spirituality, he argues, extends to 'aiding prevention, speeding recovery, and fostering equanimity in the face of ill health'; for example, research has recently demonstrated the clear role of spirituality in protecting terminally ill cancer patients from 'end of life despair'.[2]

Spirituality and music

It can be argued that music is *the* universal connecting feature of humanity. Our entrance into the world at birth is heralded by a 'song', which is responded to regardless of culture and place, and this song provides access to all our needs in the first moments and days of life. Foods protection, love, warmth, reassurance, all are satisfied through the production of sound gradually modulated to provide a universal language, which precedes speech. Acculturation can ensure that this song is *central* to life (as in many African cultures)[8] or results in it being *peripheral* where responsibility is given to 'musicians' (as in the Western European performance tradition):

> Spend any Sunday in a South African township and you will understand that a culture in which singing is upheld as a necessary function to keep body, soul and faith intact, is a healthier one; people from all generations, from grand parents to grand children, sing together, all uniting to express their faith. It's the communal singing that unites them in a very powerful very uplifting way. Singing is not a miracle cure for the world's ills, but it's one kind of medication that can have remarkable results.[8] (p.32)

Given the commonality of music among all peoples (and yet acknowledging the different place *musicking* occupies in different cultures), it is no surprise that we refer to music at times as a *universal* language. Music provides a means by which we can communicate with each other without reference to spoken language, transcending human-created barriers of politics, religion, ethnicity, class and gender. Music is used to stir the emotions, unite the team, encourage the faint-hearted, relieve misery, celebrate life and mourn death. Music is primordial, within us all, at the very heart of our existence, the reason why man, for millennia, has used music as a means to enhance wellbeing.

Spirituality and religion have significant associations with music. Some of the most profound and significant musical compositions in the Western musical tradition were inspired by spiritual aspirations or religious texts. Music and singing have throughout the history of Christianity at least, provided a powerful accompaniment for religious ceremony, and a vehicle for individual and collective worship. Music undoubtedly has powers to move people emotionally and to inspire and uplift spiritually – but does this necessarily mean that music and music making have the power to affect health in a meaningful way, or to make a valuable contribution to healthcare and treatment?

Before exploring these issues further, it is important to consider findings from research on what music means to people and the role music has in their lives. In a recent sociological analysis of music in everyday life, DeNora[9] has argued that:

> ...music's semiotic force – its effect upon hearing – cannot be fully specified in advance of actual reception. This is because musical affect is contingent upon the circumstances of music's appropriation; it is ... the product of 'human-music interaction' ... musical affect is constituted reflexively, in and through the practice of articulating or connecting music with other things. (p.20)

DeNora presents results from an interview study involving 52 women to show how people use music to 'regulate, elaborate and substantiate themselves as social agents', and claims that nearly every woman interviewed was explicit about music's role as an ordering device at a personal level, in 'creating, enhancing, sustaining and changing subjective, bodily and self-conceptual states'[9] (p.57).

Beatrice, one of the participants in DeNora's study, described the use of music in her family in response to disagreements and feelings of anger:

> Whenever anyone gets angry we all tend to go to our rooms and turn on the music really loud. ...I just go to my room, slam the door, play my music and just sort of feel mad for a couple more minutes... When I turn the music up real loud it fills my room, it's like I can't hear anything outside my room and just me really mad.[9] (p.62)

And Henrietta described how she used music to heighten and then release a sad emotional state:

> The Verdi Requiem is one of my favourites. That is associated with losing a baby. And I'd got to know it through my husband and it was really quite a way of grieving – I'd shut myself away in a room [she begins to cry]... It's cathartic, I think.[9] (p.64)

From such examples, DeNora concludes that music does not simply act upon individuals:

> Rather, music's 'effects' come from the ways in which individuals orient to it, how they interpret it and how they place it within their personal musical maps, with the semiotic web of music and extra-musical associations.[9] (p.68)

DeNora's contribution is important in sensitising us to the fact that in a healthcare setting music cannot be seen as 'a treatment' or 'intervention' that is somehow 'applied' in the care of patients. We have rather to consider the meaning that music has for individuals and the ways in which they wish to employ the resources of music in relation to their own circumstances – including any difficulties with health they may be experiencing. How then is music connected with the spiritual dimensions of life in the experiences of individuals? And how do individuals see the role of music in relation to their health? Some recent research studies have explored both of these issues with individuals outside of healthcare settings.

Research on spirituality, music and health

Research has highlighted the links between spiritual experiences and music from two directions.

Experiencing the spiritual

First, some studies have explored the extent to which people have experiences that they regard as spiritual. These may be described in a wide variety of ways, for example, elevating, joyful, being at one with the world, peaceful, in touch with a higher power. The studies have shown that music is often a factor associated with, or giving rise to, such experiences. Greeley,[10] for example, asked 1467 American adults the question, 'Have you ever felt as though you were very close to a powerful spiritual force that seemed to lift you out of yourself?' Just over a third answered yes, and of these respondents, just under half cited music as the most frequent trigger of such experiences. Other triggers described were prayer, the beauties of nature and quiet reflection.

Lowis[11] explored the factors associated with 'peak emotional experiences' among staff at a British university college, by asking about such experiences, for example, 'Have you ever had an experience where you were passive (such as, relaxing, listening, thinking or meditating) and felt a heightened sense of clarity, reality, insight, revelation, solution or totally enveloping joy?' Among 364 participants, just over three-quarters reported experiencing a peak emotional experience under such conditions, and music was identified as the most common antecedent of these experiences by over half of respondents (55%).

Lowis concluded from his study that:

> In fact music may have a special role: it is a form of non-verbal communication which is said to appeal directly to the 'soul'[12] and form a bridge for us to the inner (spiritual) world.[13] (Lowis, p.51)

Both these studies are of interest in showing that some people do not acknowledge 'spiritual' experiences in their lives, and among those who do, not all of them regard music as a significant conduit for such experience. This suggests that only certain people would see music as a source of spiritual support in the context of coping with health problems.

Experiences of listening to and participating in music

A second group of studies has explored personal experiences of listening to and participating in music. These studies have highlighted the widespread emotional significance of music and, more specifically for some, the links with spiritual beliefs and experience.

Listening to recorded music

Lowis and Hughes[14] explored the emotional and spiritual dimensions of listening to recorded music – both sacred and secular – with groups of elderly people. A number of extracts of music were played to elderly participants and they were asked to rate them in terms of the feelings they evoked. Most participants found the selections restful and evocative for memories and thoughtfulness. In addition, those participants found to have a more spiritual outlook on life, were more likely to rate both kinds of music highly for their qualities of reverence and spirituality.

Participating in choirs

Clift and Hancox[15] asked members of a UK university college choral society (approximately 100 members) rehearsing Rutter's *Requiem* and Vivaldi's *Gloria* to complete a simple questionnaire asking whether they believed that singing had benefits for them – physically, emotionally, socially and spiritually – and to describe what they were. The majority of participants believed they benefited socially (87%) and emotionally (75%), over half believed they benefited physically (58%) and just under half felt some spiritual benefit (49%). Interestingly, the language employed to describe spiritual benefits revealed a considerable overlap with descriptions of emotional benefit and some aspects of social benefit, with participants referring to feeling positive, happier and less stressed, and experiencing therapeutic benefits and a sense of unity or a bond with the group as a whole. Requests to explain spiritual benefits did, however, give rise to distinctive accounts such as describing singing as uplifting, refreshing the soul, enhancing spiritual or religious beliefs and having 'intangible effects which are difficult to explain'. Interesting comments also came from choir members emphasising what they saw as the intimate connections between the physical and spiritual aspects of life:

> It's good for one's soul and what's good for your soul is good for your body.

> If your physical side is related to your spiritual side then it can do only good. Healthy mind, healthy body, etc.

In a second study, Clift and Hancox[15] used a structured questionnaire developed on the basis of choir members' previous descriptions, and 'spiritual' statements prompted wider endorsement than those of a more clearly 'religious' nature.

Community singing groups with elderly people

In 1989, Hillman[16] set up the community arts project *Call That Singing!* – a year-long programme designed to encourage participation in Glasgow's celebrations as European Capital of Culture 1990. The project proved so successful, particularly with older people, that it continues to flourish. *Call That Singing!* encourages people of all ages and abilities, social and cultural backgrounds, and particularly those who think they can't sing, to participate in a mass singing group which offers a programme of fun rehearsals and shows.

The impetus for Hillman's questionnaire-based study came about through observations of people involved in *Call That Singing!* and their articulation of the perceived positive effects on their general health and wellbeing. The research project was set up to determine whether there is any evidence to support the general view that 'singing is good for you'.

The results clearly showed that participants perceived a variety of benefits to mental health, including the following.

- Marked improvements in perceptions of emotional wellbeing, particularly among those who were widowed; participatory singing was perceived to be pleasurable, fun, uplifting and relaxing, and helped to counter depression, grief and concerns with physical health.
- Improvements in social life; *Call That Singing!* gave people the opportunity to get out of the house, meet new people, make new friends and develop a network from which to socialise beyond rehearsal nights.
- Improvements to self-confidence, which manifested in participants' pleasure in their improved singing skills and abilities to perform for others.
- Improvements in singing skills and general understanding of music increased self-confidence and led to increased visits to arts and cultural events.
- Improvements to general quality of life confirmed the view that participatory singing helped to combat the potentially negative effects of ageing, along with the debilitating effects of bereavement, widowhood, declining health and isolation.

Choral singing and homeless men

Bailey and Davidson[17,18] report a fascinating study evaluating the significance of a choral singing project established for homeless men in Quebec. *The Homeless Choir* was established in December 1996 through the efforts of a young man who volunteered at a busy soup kitchen. He felt that his volunteer work didn't really help the men he was working with to change their lives in a positive direction, and from his own experience of choral singing had the idea that forming a choir with homeless men might provide a way to help the homeless help themselves. Starting with only three members, the choir grew and eventually stabilised at around 20 members.

Seven of the 19 members of the choir (aged 45 to 59) were interviewed to explore the contribution made by group singing to the positive changes that occurred. Several themes consistently emerged from a content analysis of the interviews.

- Active participation in singing appeared to alleviate depression.
- Choir members believed that singing restores mental and physical balance.
- A correlation was perceived between emotional stability and the time spent in the choir.
- Reciprocity between the choir and the audience appeared to provide personal validation and may have improved social interaction skills.
- Participation in the choir resulted in more appropriate interactions among the choir members.
- The mental engagement required to learn and perform the repertoire appeared to direct attention away from disturbing internal thoughts and to promote ordered thinking.

The benefits of choral singing for homeless men are illustrated by the following comment from one of the interviewees:

> For me it's very therapeutic, as before coming here I was in very bad shape emotionally. The emotional part of it [the singing] will last eight to 20 hours, you know, and that's worth a lot of money. These days I suffer from arthritis in the knees, but the minute the music starts I don't feel my arthritis anymore. For me it's a drug. (Raoul,[17] p.240)

Bailey and Davidson[17] argue that accounts such as this provide 'evidence that suggests that singing promotes physical and emotional balance and may provide a period of alleviation from a variety of physical and emotional symptoms' (p.245).

Music, medicine and healthcare

The idea that music can have a significant role in healing ailments of mind and body has deep historical roots in Western culture[19] and is endorsed within many non-Western cultural traditions.[20] A considerable body of recent research has explored the therapeutic use of music for a wide range of physical, neurophysiological and psychosocial problems, as well as the role of music to alleviate pain and reduce stress and anxiety in the contexts of medical and surgical procedures.[21,22] Research has also explored the effects of listening to music and active participation in music making on objective indicators of physiological, neurological and immunological function.[23–29]

Hallam,[30] in a review of literature on the power of music, reaches a number of general conclusions, and the following key points from her summary highlight important conclusions emerging from the literature.

- Music is powerful at the level of the social group because it facilitates communication which goes beyond words, induces shared emotional reactions and supports the development of group identity.
- Music is powerful at the individual level because it can induce multiple responses – physiological, movement, mood, emotional, cognitive and behavioural.
- Music has powerful therapeutic effects, which can be achieved through listening or active music making.
- Music can promote relaxation, alleviate anxiety and pain, promote appropriate behaviour in vulnerable groups and enhance the quality of life of those who are beyond medical help.
- People can use music in their lives to manipulate their moods, alleviate the boredom of tedious tasks and create environments appropriate for particular social events.
- The easy availability of music in everyday life is encouraging individuals to use music to optimise their sense of wellbeing.

Similarly, Staricoff[22] has recently reviewed the extensive medical literature on the effects of the arts, mainly music, on different healthcare specialities, both for in-patients and for those attending outpatient departments, and highlights encouraging findings in areas of cancer care, pain management, mental health treatments, surgical procedures of all kinds and work with Alzheimer's patients, to name but a few specialist areas of care.

Four organisations bringing music into healthcare

The idea that musical activities and singing can have benefits in healthcare settings – for patients and for staff too – is at the core of the work of several charitable organisations and projects currently operating in the UK. The aims of these initiatives are described briefly, together with some of the feedback they have received from their activities.

Music in Hospitals

Music in Hospitals[31] was established in 1948 and now presents in the region of 4000 live concerts every year throughout the UK, reaching some 120 000 patients, residents and clients. It aims to improve the quality of life of adults and children in hospitals through the benefits of live music, and organises concerts given by professional musicians in healthcare settings across the UK. They work with children, elderly people, the terminally ill, people with disabilities and those with mental health problems. For those with life-threatening illnesses, *Music in Hospitals* believes that a concert offers 'comfort and emotional release'. For older people, they suggest 'memories are revived and all kinds of emotions are released' (*Music in Hospitals* website). The pleasure that these concerts can bring is more powerfully conveyed by pictures than words (Figure 12.1).

(a)

(b)

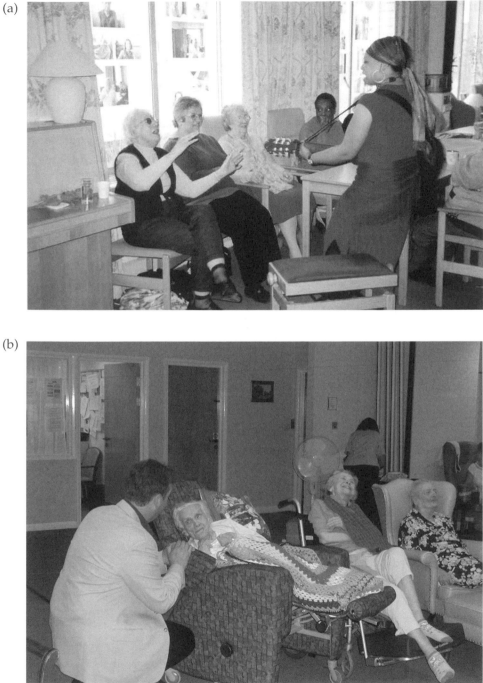

© *Music in Hospitals.*

Figure 12.1 Images of *Music in Hospitals* musicians entertaining elderly patients. (a) 'Some particular patients (normally very withdrawn) came out of their shells and you could see it in their faces, the delight of being sung to and being part of an activity'; (b) 'One resident who hardly smiles or interacts with staff was beaming all through the performance'. With permission from *Music in Hospitals.*

Live Music Now!

Live Music Now![32] was founded in 1977 by the violinist Yehudi Menuhin and Ian Stoutzker. It aims to use the expertise of professional musicians to help people access the joy of live music in venues such as schools for children with special needs, centres for adults with physical and learning disabilities, homes for older people, young offenders institutions, prisons, hospitals and hospices. The focus is not simply on musicians performing:

> There are always opportunities for members of the audience to get involved in ways which are appropriate such as, musical games, asking and answering questions, singing, dancing, playing percussion and conducting. Whether they wish to listen quietly or to participate actively these experiences are exhilarating, educational and therapeutic. (*Live Music Now!* website)

Jessie's Fund

Jessie's Fund[33] was established as a registered charity in April 1995 with the aim of helping sick children in all areas of the UK through the therapeutic use of music. Its major concern has been to establish and expand the availability and scope of therapeutic music in children's hospices. The achievements of Jessie's Fund over the past 10 years have been considerable in developing the role of music in children's hospices, and it has extended its work with children to a range of other healthcare and community settings.

Singing Medicine

Singing Medicine[34,35] is the most recently established project devised by Ex Cathedra Education and Birmingham Children's Hospital. It aims to use a range of singing activities to develop children's musicianship, vocal performance and skills as well as personal, social, health and emotional skills.

Serious attention is being given to evaluating this project, and a report is due to appear in late 2005. So far, there are encouraging signs that singing activities have important benefits for children in hospital – an environment that is often associated with negative emotions of fear, anxiety, pain and boredom:

> Above all singing is fun. Singing activities also offer better social inclusion on the hospital wards, deep breathing to aid recovery and can help prevent infection, coping mechanisms and distraction techniques.[35] (p.27)

Music, spirituality and healthcare

The reviews by Hallam[30] and Staricoff,[22] and the four projects described, undoubtedly demonstrate that music can be used to promote a personal sense of wellbeing, pleasure and social interaction in patients and so enhance the quality of the healthcare environment. To what extent, however, is music valuable specifically in supporting spiritual dimensions of care? A feature of the practical projects outlined is that they generally appear to involve music within group settings, and so the character of engagement and emotional expression tends to be both public and upbeat. Conversely, serious engagement with and expression of spiritual issues may be regarded as being more personal and private, and more likely to emerge in one-to-one encounters. Furthermore, while all of the projects are keen to emphasise the 'therapeutic' dimension of their work, only one speaks specifically about 'music therapy' and the work of music therapists (*Jessie's Fund*), and music therapy may provide a more appropriate context for spiritual issues to emerge.

To explore this further, the reviews of previous research by Hallam[30] and Staricoff[22] were searched using relevant terms based on the facets of 'spiritual, religious and personal beliefs' identified by the WHOQOL project (*see* p.151):

- religion, religious
- spirit, spiritual, spirituality
- meaningfulness, purposefulness
- awe, wonder
- wholeness, holistic
- inner peace, inner world
- hope, optimism
- faith
- transcendent, transcendental.

This proved surprisingly unproductive, as few of these words and phrases were used in either review in relation to any context or art form. In Staricoff, the word 'spirit' occurred twice, 'hope' once and 'inner world' once; in Hallam, 'religion/ religious' occurred twice, 'spirit' twice, 'holistic' three times and 'transcendent' once. The only source identified that has particular relevance to 'spirituality' is an article by Schroeder[36] describing the field of 'music-thanatology'.

Music-thanatology

Schroeder[36] describes music-thanatology as a palliative medical modality employing prescriptive music to tend the complex physical and spiritual needs of the dying. Although based on the tradition of 'Infirmary music' developed within French monastic medicine in eleventh-century Cluny, music-thanatology does not espouse any particular religious tradition, but is nevertheless concerned with the possibility of a 'blessed death' and the notion that conscious dying can contribute to the fullness of life. Music-thanatology practitioners deliver prescriptive music through playing a small four-octave harp and singing in bedside vigils serving the dying at home, and in hospital and hospice settings.

The origins of music-thanology are described by Cassidy[37] in Box 12.1. A video demonstration of music-thanatology is available,[38] and reviews of the film include the following comment:

> As a hospice nurse for 15 years, I found Ms Schroeder-Sheker insightful and 'right on' target with her observations of the goals of a 'good death'. Focusing on a safe sanctuary for the patient and their loved ones, including the peaceful atmosphere created by music, allows the patient and their loved ones to speak those important words of reconciliation, love, and ultimate joy that the joining of their lives has brought.[38]

To date, only one study designed to assess the effectiveness of prescriptive harp music on selected palliative care outcomes has been reported.[39] Sixty-five patients were administered a 25- to 95-minute intervention of prescriptive harp music. Two certified music-thanatologists collected vital signs (respiration rate, pulse rate and rhythm) before the vigil began and again following the vigil. Observational indicators (wakefulness, agitation and depth of breath) were also assessed. Results from this study provide evidence that a prescriptive vigil conducted by a trained music-thanatologist may have positive effects on dying patients. Patients were more likely to experience decreased levels of agitation and decreased levels of wakefulness (the patient was in a more restful state), while also being able to breathe more slowly and deeply with less effort. Freeman concluded that her findings suggest that healthcare settings and practitioners, as well as family members, should consider music-thanatology as a form of palliative care for dying patients.

Box 12.1   The origins of music-thanatology[37]

He was a lonely old man, a combative patient facing death. She was an undergraduate music student earning college money as an orderly in a nursing home. Their lives were about to intersect and change in a profound and mysterious way.

Entering the room where the man lay frightened and dying, his last breaths rattling in his chest, the orderly, Therese Schroeder-Sheker, was moved to make this man's death a blessed one. She said his name, held him and sang the hymns 'Ubi Caritas', 'Salve Regina' and 'The Mass of the Angels' in her clear soprano voice. And then, Schroeder-Sheker recalls, 'The desperate thrashing stopped. The death rattle quieted. This man who had a history of pushing everyone away actually trusted me, rested into me, and slowly, because of the quiet singing, we began to breathe together. When I walked home that night after he died, I understood his passage as a kind of birth.'

Since that first vigil at the bedside of a dying patient more than 30 years ago, Schroeder-Sheker – a musician, educator and CUA (Catholic University of America) artist- and clinician-in-residence – has sung and played her harp at thousands of bedsides. She has pioneered the field of music-thanatology, the physical and spiritual care of the dying via 'prescriptive music', and through the Chalice of Repose Project she founded, has trained scores of other music-thanatologists who now work in the United States, Canada, the Netherlands, Israel and Japan. But she's never forgotten that first patient. 'That moment of combined song and prayer now seems crucial. The music was not a form of distraction therapy,' she says. 'It had become a genuine medicine.'

Final reflections

The significance of the spiritual dimension of life for health is widely acknowledged, and this chapter has attempted to consider the place of music in the links between spirituality, health and healthcare. Music has deep roots in the evolution of the human psyche; it serves together with language to distinguish us from all other species. We are born with an innate capacity to respond to music, and throughout life music has a special place for most people. Music has a profound capacity to connect with and express our emotions, and can open up a world of experience and beauty, which goes beyond the mundane and the banal realities of everyday life. It can therefore provide a powerful resource in promoting health in a holistic sense, embracing physical, social and mental wellbeing.

It is important, however, to exercise caution in claiming too much for music in the links between spirituality and healthcare. While it may be true that every individual has spiritual needs, in the sense that meaning and purpose in life are essential for personal and emotional wellbeing, it is clearly the case that many individuals, at least in Western societies, would not describe themselves 'spiritual' and fewer still would profess strongly held religious beliefs. As we have seen, Greeley's research[10] on 'spiritual' experiences indicates that only approximately a third of adults reported such experiences. Similarly, while the connections between music and spirituality are undoubtedly strong at a cultural level, it doesn't necessarily mean that the connections are strong for every individual. Again, although Greeley found that music was the most common trigger for 'spiritual' experiences, about half of those reporting such experiences did not mention music as giving rise to them. Similar points could be made in relation to the other studies reviewed above: music and spirituality are linked for some people – but equally some spiritual people do not tie their beliefs or experiences to music, just as some people devoted to music may not regard it as giving access to the world of the spirit.

These points should be borne in mind when considering the role of music in the spiritual dimensions of healthcare. There is no doubt that musical activity and singing can make a tremendous contribution in healthcare settings, in improving the quality of the environment and promoting personal and social wellbeing. Organisations such as *Music in Hospitals* could not have continued to thrive over many years if their contributions did not consistently generate the enthusiasm among patients and health professionals alike, which is reflected in the feedback and images given above. This does not necessarily mean, however, that the music they offer plays an important role in addressing patients' spiritual needs. The fact that a search of the reviews by Hallam[30] and Staricoff[22] identified little reference to specifically 'spiritual' concerns also indicates that this issue has attracted little attention in the social science and medical research literature. Clearly, the links between music, spirituality and healthcare should be explored further, with a more sensitive focusing on the circumstances and experiences of individual patients.

References

1   Culliford L (2002) Spirituality and clinical care. *British Medical Journal*. **325**: 1434–5.
2   McClain CS, Rosenfield B, Breitbart W (2003) Effect of spiritual well-being on end-of-life despair in terminally-ill cancer patients. *The Lancet*. **361**: 1603–7.
3   Potts RG (2004) Spirituality, religion, and the experience of illness. In: Camic P, Knight S (eds) *Clinical Handbook of Health Psychology: a practical guide to effective interventions*. Hogrefe & Huber, Cambridge.
4   World Health Organization (1948) The WHO definition of health is to be found in the *Preamble to the Constitution of the World Health Organization* as adopted by the International Health Conference, New York, 19–22 June 1946; signed on 22 July 1946 by the representatives of 61 States (Official Records of the World Health Organization, no. 2, p.100) and entered into force on 7 April 1948.
5   Power M, Harper A, Bullinger M and The World Health Organization Quality of Life Group (1999) The World Health Organization WHOQOL-100: tests of the universality of

quality of life in 15 different cultural groups worldwide. *Health Psychology*. **18**(5): 495–505.

6   World Health Organization (2002) *WHOQOL-SRPB Users Manual: scoring and coding for the WHOQOL SRPB field-test instrument*. Mental Health Evidence and Research, Department of Mental Health and Substance Dependence. World Health Organization, Geneva.

7   Koenig HK, McCullough ME, Larson DB (2001) *Handbook of Religion and Health*. Oxford University Press, Oxford.

8   Digby S (1999) Voices Foundation. *BBC Music Magazine*. **September**: 40.

9   DeNora T (2002) *Music in Everyday Life*. Cambridge University Press, Cambridge.

10 Greeley AM (1974) *Ecstasy, A Way of Knowing*. Prentice Hall, Englewood Cliffs, NJ.

11 Lowis MJ (1998) Music and peak experiences: an empirical study. *Mankind Quarterly*. **39**(2): 203–24.

12 James J (1993) *The Music of the Spheres*. Little Brown, London.

13 Lowis MJ (2003) Peak emotional experiences and their antecedents: a survey of staff at a British University College. *The Korean Journal of Thinking & Problem Solving*. **13**(2): 41–53.

14 Lowis MJ, Hughes J (1997) A comparison of the effects of sacred and secular music on elderly people. *Journal of Psychology*. **13**(1): 45–55.

15 Clift SM, Hancox G (2001) The perceived benefits of singing: findings from preliminary surveys of a university college choral society. *Journal of the Royal Society for the Promotion of Health*. **121**(4): 248–56.

16 Hillman S (2002) Participatory singing for older people: a perception of benefit. *Health Education*. **102**(4): 32–40.

17 Bailey BA, Davidson JW (2002) Adaptive characteristics of group singing: perceptions from members of a choir for homeless men. *Musicae Scientiae*. **6**(2): 221–56.

18 Bailey BA, Davidson JW (2002) Amateur group singing as a therapeutic instrument. *Nordic Journal of Music Therapy*. **12**(1): 18–32.

19 Weldin C, Eagle C (1991) An historical overview of music and medicine. In: Maranto CD (ed.) *Applications of Music to Medicine*. National Association for Music Therapy, Washington, pp.73–84.

20 Gouk P (ed.) (2000) *Musical Healing in Cultural Contexts*. Ashgate, Aldershot.

21 Maranto CD (ed.) (1991) *Applications of Music to Medicine*. National Association for Music Therapy, Washington.

22 Staricoff RL (2004) *Arts in Health: a review of the medical literature*. Research Report 36. Arts Council, London.

23 Krumhansl CL (1997) An exploratory study of musical emotions and psychophysiology. *Canadian Journal of Experimental Psychology*. **51**(4): 336–52.

24 McCraty R, Atkinson M, Rein G *et al.* (1996) Music enhances the effect of positive emotional states on salivary IgA. *Stress Medicine*. **12**: 167–75.

25 Charnetski CJ, Brennan FX, Harrison JF (1998) Effect of music and auditory stimuli on secretory immunoglobulin A (IgA). *Perceptual and Motor Skills*. **87**: 1163–70.

26 Beck RJ, Cesario TC, Yousefi A *et al.* (1999) Choral singing, performance perception, and immune system changes in salivary immunoglobulin A and cortisol. *Music Perception*. **18**: 87–106.

27 Bittman BB, Berk LS, Felten DL *et al.* (2001) Composite effects of group drumming music therapy on modulation of neuroendrocrine-immune parameters in normal subjects. *Alternative Therapy, Health and Medicine*. **7**(1): 38–47.

28 Panksepp J, Bernatzky G (2002) Emotional sounds and the brain: the neuro-affective foundations of musical appreciation. *Behavioural Processes*. **60**: 133–55.

29 Kreutz G, Bongard S, Rohrmann S *et al.* (2004) Effects of choir singing or listening on secretory immunoglobulin A, cortisol, and emotional state. *Journal of Behavioral Medicine*. **27**(6): 623–35.

30 Hallam S (2001) *The Power of Music*. Performing Rights Society, London. Available through the Performing Rights Society website: www.mcps-prs-alliance.co.uk (accessed 17 July 2005).

31 *Music in Hospitals* www.music-in-hospitals.org.uk

32 *Live Music Now!* www.livemusicnow.org

33 *Jessie's Fund* www.jessiesfund.org.uk

34   *Singing Medicine* www.creative-remedies.org.uk/casestudies.asp

35   Youth Music (2005) Healthy option: this singing project for sick children is just what the doctor ordered. *Feedback: Your Essential Youth Music Update.* **1**: 26–7.

36   Schroeder T (1994) Music for the dying: a personal account of the new field of music-thanatology – history, theories, and clinical narratives. *Journal of Holistic Nursing.* **12**(1): 83–99.

37   Cassidy A (2004) Helping patients die a good death. *The Catholic University of America Online Newspaper.* **5 November**. Available at: http://inside.cua.edu/041105/story2.cfm (accessed 17 July 2005).

38   Schroeder-Sheker T (1997) *Chalice of Repose.* Sounds True, VHS. (Available through www.amazon.com (accessed 17 July 2005).

39   Freeman L (2004) *Music thanatology: prescriptive harp music as palliative care for the dying patient.* Unpublished PhD thesis, Health Sciences Center, University of Utah.

Conclusion

Wendy Greenstreet

The complex nature of the concept of spirituality has been reflected throughout this book as one that cannot be conveyed in a single definition. It is an abstract phenomenon that cannot be reduced to a single form. Its situation within health and social contexts is found in its description as part of holistic care. This description presupposes that every person has a spiritual dimension. How well this dimension of a person is developed is dependent on many factors, including cognitive, moral, personality development, age and socialisation. For some, this dimension may remain dormant, unacknowledged and effectively non-existent, and so not be part of their 'world-view'. However, others may reach a level of spiritual development resulting in a selflessness and vision that acts as an inspiration to the world at large. Most people who reflect on their own spiritual stance find themselves somewhere between these two extremes.

Descriptions of the phenomenon spirituality can 'loosely' be grouped as religious or sacred or secular. Each of these categories provides a different means of approaching life's ultimate questions. Circumstances that render individuals in need of health and social care may precipitate such questioning that seeks to know 'why?'. There is an increased acknowledgement of spirituality as a perspective of care by government and professional regulatory bodies. This is accompanied by some advocating the need for a professional rhetoric of spirituality to ensure that the spiritual is valued alongside the scientific. This rhetoric needs to reflect spirituality as a 'cocktail' of varying strengths of components of religious, sacred and secular possibilities for each individual, rather than stereotyping clients/patients into one of three polarised groupings.

Spirituality needs to be part of a professional's world-view if they are to assess the need for, and contribute to, spiritual care. Some initial assessment of personal spiritual stance is an important requirement in participating in this aspect of care, but developing spiritual intelligence provides a more robust preparation. Assessment tools can be used to 'do' a 'spiritual assessment' and provide data of outward expressions of spirituality. However, a richer awareness of a patient's spirituality is more likely to emerge from within an established rapport between client/patient and professional in the throes of delivering psychosocial and physical care, rather than a contrived separate assessment of spiritual need.

Spiritual care can fundamentally be conceived as having two facets. First, and the most easily understood, are practical activities that we can 'do' for those in our care. These include facilitating client/patient access to the means for them to fulfil their own spiritual needs. Knowledge of the historical and philosophical developments behind the term 'religion' should help professionals understand commonalities and differences between religions of faith and experience, rather than viewing religions as either good or bad, familiar or alien. This knowledge promotes tolerance through the understanding of the potential different perspectives clients/patients might have in relation to the meaning of their ill health or difficulties. A greater awareness of the meaning and significance of religious rituals in promoting spiritual wellbeing should spur professionals on to make arrangements for religious practices to be possible. Professional carers also need to have a fundamental understanding of cultural and religious requirements of world religions and ethnic minorities so that they can offer practical support, for example, in relation to diet, physical examination and care of the dying.

Supplementary and/or alternative sources of activity that potentially contribute to spiritual health are creative therapies that include music, art and spiritual counselling. Blackthorn Trust exemplifies the benefits of how specialists offering creative activities alongside conventional practice promote spiritual wellbeing in those with serious or long-term health problems. The benefits to wellbeing of listening to and participating in music are clearly demonstrated by, for example, Music in Hospitals. If listening to music is identified as particularly uplifting by a client/patient, most professionals could arrange for this to be possible. However, access to music-thanatology that provides spiritual benefit for the dying would certainly require referral to specialist performers.

Spirituality is a complex phenomenon and so the provision of spiritual care is not the prerogative of any one profession. However, it is important that professionals understand their personal and professional limits in relation to contributing to spiritual care. Referring clients/patients to others who can offer specialist support in fulfilling their identified spiritual needs is an act of care in itself if, for example, specific religious support, creative therapy or spiritual counselling is needed.

The second way in which spiritual care can be conveyed is through authentic relationship. Existential philosophy has been used to illustrate the notion of selfhood and being with others that exemplify authenticity. Sharing self in authentic relationship reflects the art of care. Advanced communication skills, including attentive listening, intuition and confidence in picking up client/patient cues that allude to intimate matters of a spiritual nature, moves the professional's presence of physically 'being there' to psychologically 'being with' those in their care. On occasion, the expression of need and its fulfilment are achieved simply by the professional carer sharing their presence in 'being with' the client/patient at that moment.

Hope is central to spiritual care, conveying a sense of future that contributes to the purpose of life ahead. Its intangible essence and dynamic nature make a qualitative approach to assessment of hope the most appropriate. This needs to be centred on a rapport that facilitates a trusting relationship. Understanding the process of hope is helpful to professional carers in demonstrating how they can support clients/patients in setting goal(s) to achieve particular hope(s) in overcoming the threat that difficulty and ill health presents. Similarly, hope-promoting strategies are helpful in supporting clients/patients to generate more generalised hope. Hope cannot be given, it can only be maintained or inspired. Authentic relationship is the vehicle for achieving this.

Professionals who share themselves in the spiritual care of others will themselves need support. Spirituality concerns a sense of connection with ourselves and others within the contexts in which we live and work. Reflective practice, clinical supervision and mentoring are options to provide staff with appropriate support. Organisations that encourage a sense of meaning and purpose in work and invest in an ambience of positive relationships are more likely to nourish the spirits of their staff.

Education provides a forum to raise professional awareness of the debates surrounding spirituality in health and social care contexts. In providing a space that is supportive in allowing professionals to be themselves, and free from the restrictions of practice settings, educational forums can utilise 'the human ability to deal with experience by creating model situations and to master reality by experiment and planning' (Erikson 1965, cited,[1] p.52). In this way, questions of what is spirituality in health and social care contexts, and how can the challenges of the provision of spiritual care for those in need be met, can be explored. Discussion using anecdotes from practice within multiprofessional groups provide an ideal opportunity to explore issues inter-professionally and generate a shared rhetoric of spirituality for health and social care professionals.

Reference

1 Grainger R (2003) *Group Spirituality, A Workshop Approach.* Brunner–Routledge, Hove.

Appendix

Case study: dying as a Tibetan Buddhist

Burkhard Scherer

This example should demonstrate how important it is to be aware of and respect differing spiritual practices and needs Within Buddhist cultures, death and birth (re-becoming) are part of the cycle of 'wandering' (*samsara*) the world of suffering, fuelled by cause and effect (*karma*). The ultimate cause of suffering is our incapability to see 'things as they are': confusion/ignorance (*avidya*) and attachment/desire (*trishna, raga*). The absolute reality is enlightenment, highest joy.

According to Tibetan Buddhism,[1,2] the process of dying entails the gradual dissolving of the five gross elements.

- **Earth** (solidity) dissolves into water: the body loses strength, the patient begins to feel disorientated.
- **Water** (fluids) dissolves into fire: body loses control over fluids, the patient becomes dehydrated.
- **Fire** (warmth) dissolves into air/wind: body loses warmth, the patient starts shivering, feeling cold.
- **Air**/wind (breath) dissolves into space: the breath activity becomes slow and decreases.
- **Space** dissolves into consciousness itself: total immobility of patient, last breath.

Now the person is clinically dead, but according to Tibetan Buddhist tradition, this is just the beginning of the dying process proper, taking around 20–30 minutes after the clinical death.

- **First 10–15 minutes**: the white, male energy descends from the crown of the head through the central axis of the body (central energy channel) towards the heart centre. Thirty-three forms of disturbing emotions resulting from anger disappear.
- **Following 10–15 minutes**: the red, female energy ascends from the sexual energy point, one hand wide below the navel (prostrate, G-point), towards the heart centre. Forty forms of disturbing emotions resulting from desire disappear.
- **Point of union**: the white and red energy melt together in the heart centre. Seven forms of disturbing emotions resulting from ignorance disappear.

After that, the dying person normally becomes 'unconscious' and 'awakes' after 68–72 hours: the *chönyi bardo* (chos nyid bar do; intermediate state between death and rebirth/re-becoming) begins and lasts a maximum of 49 days.

For those initiated into the meditation of the *Bardo Thödol* (bar do thos grol, 'Tibetan Book of the Dead'), the experiences of different Buddha aspects occur.[3]

There is also a specific Tibetan Buddhist meditation during the process of dying called *phowa* (pho ba), in which the dying person transfers their consciousness through the crown of the head into a state of mind outside suffering and confusion, a so called 'pure land'. A qualified Buddhist teacher or practitioner can assist the dying person during this meditation. If the dying person has not practised the *phowa* meditation before, they can, for instance, focus at the moment of death on the red Buddha of Limitless Light (*Amitabha*):

> Above the crown of my head, there is the Buddha of Limitless Light shining like a mountain of rubies in the light of 1000 suns. He is everything I wish for and trust in. There I want to go.
> (Recitation of the mantra: OM AMI DEWA HRIH)

This specific spiritual setting carries interesting implications. When dealing with Tibetan Buddhists in palliative care, the medical personnel can care for the specific spiritual needs of the patients at different stages.

1 The patient should be as free from pain and as conscious as possible at the same time.
2 The mantra OM MANI PEME HUNG is beneficial for all sentient beings and can be used with ill people (more specific mantras, e.g. Medicine Buddha, need transmission by a qualified Buddhist teacher (Lama)).
3 A Buddhist minister, meditation master or Buddhist friends should be able to be present; the Lama should at least be notified, especially when the last breath took place.
4 No wailing/moaning should disturb the dying process (to avoid the generation of confusion and attachment within the dying person).
5 The mantra OM AMI DEWA HRIH is very beneficial for dying people once the terminal process is irreversible (especially after the last breath): say it inwardly or outwardly, whisper it in the dying person's ear, blow it on the tips of your fingers and then place it gently on the crown of the dying person's head, etc.
6 Once the dying process has started and especially for the 30 minutes after the last breath, the person should not be touched, moved or disturbed in any other way. This is a critical time and a rare opportunity for the dying to realise enlightenment.

References

1 Lama Lodö (1982) *Bardo Teachings: the way of death and rebirth*. Snow Lion, Ithaca, NY.
2 Sogyal Rinpoche (1992) *The Tibetan Book of Living and Dying*. Harper Collins Publishers, San Francisco, CA.
3 Fremantle F, Chögyam Trungpa (1975) *The Tibetan Book of the Dead: the great liberation through hearing in the Bardo*. Shambala, Berkeley, CA.

Index

Page numbers in *italics* refer to figures or boxes.